COURTS AND
MODERN MEDICINE

COURTS AND
MODERN MEDICINE

By

ANTHONY CHAMPAGNE, Ph.D.

Associate Professor
Political Science Department
The University of Texas at Dallas
Richardson, Texas

and

ROSEMARY N. DAWES, M.S.N., M.A.

Dawes Consulting Associates
Allen, Texas

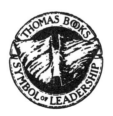

CHARLES C THOMAS • PUBLISHER

Springfield • Illinois • U.S.A.

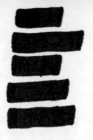

Published and Distributed Throughout the World by

CHARLES C THOMAS • PUBLISHER

2600 South First Street

Springfield, Illinois 62717

© *1983 by* CHARLES C THOMAS • PUBLISHER

ISBN 0-398-4834-74834-7

Library of Congress Catalog Card Number: 82-25628

With THOMAS BOOKS *careful attention is given to all details of manufacturing and*
design. It is the Publisher's desire to present books that are satisfactory as to their physical
qualities and artistic possibilities and appropriate for their particular use. THOMAS
BOOKS *will be true to those laws of quality that assure a good name and good will.*

Printed in the United States of America
Q-R-3

Library of Congress Cataloging in Publication Data

Champagne, Anthony.
    Courts and modern medicine.

    Bibliography: p.
    Includes index.
    1. Medical laws and legislation--United States--Cases.
2. Judicial process--United States--Cases.   I. Daws,
Rosemary N. II. Title. [DNLM: 1. Legislation, Medi-
cal--United States--Cases. W 32.5 AA1 C4c]
KF3821.A7C33   1983   344.73'041'0264   82-25628
ISBN 0-398-04834-7   347.304410264

To our families

PREFACE

COURTS in America have become increasingly involved in the making of public policy. Evidence of judicial activism and policymaking is found in a wide variety of areas that include education, reapportionment, equal treatment, and, increasingly, medicine. In part, activism is a matter of choice for judges. They may purposefully lower the self-imposed barriers to judicial policymaking in order to have an impact upon society. Additionally, in our litigious society, judges are called upon to solve problems that in the past would have been dealt with informally or may never have been dealt with at all. It may also be the case that courts are more and more called upon to deal with questions that the political branches can not or will not handle.[1]

There is no area of judicial policymaking that raises more profound problems than medicine. In this area, the courts must try to establish and reflect fundamental societal values. These values concern the meaning of death and the meaning of life. When, for example, may it be said that death is preferable to life? At what point, if any, may society infringe upon an individual's reproductive choices? To what extent may individuals assert a right to health care? May patients claim a right to seek alternative treatments? When may others make health choices for minors or incompetents?

In some cases it is the courts that must deal with personal tragedies and construct a legal justification to resolve a problem. Many such cases never get to the courts. Informal decisions of physicians, patients, and patients' families probably continue to resolve most of these problems. On those occasions when the courts do become involved, however, values are stated as societal values, and precedents are established to govern society's future choices. Since court decisions are often made with reference to concepts of rights, value compromises or changes of mind become especially difficult once the courts become involved.[2]

---

[1]For example, see Horowitz, Donald: *The Courts and Social Policy.*. Washington, D.C., Brookings, 1977.
[2]Ibid., pp. 34-35.

vii

This book is an effort to pull together a number of judicial choices in several significant areas of medicine. An introductory essay begins each chapter, and questions are raised to assist the reader in a personal assessment of the judicial decision.

This collection of cases is not designed to examine all legal-medical questions, nor are all cases or viewpoints examined in each issue area. One should not read these cases to find definitive answers or settled matters of law. Rather, this casebook is an effort to present the value judgments of a variety of courts in such a way that the reader may consider some of the ways important legal-medical issues have been addressed and so that the reader may determine the appropriateness of that decision.[3]

The book should prove useful to those in the medical community. The legal community should also find this book useful as should policy scientists, philosophers, students, and lay persons concerned about the interaction between the courts and modern medicine.

A final note about the cases. The cases have been edited — sometimes extensively. Three asterisks separating paragraphs indicate that one or more paragraphs have been deleted. A series of periods indicate that part of a sentence or several sentences in a paragraph have been deleted. Headings and subheadings within the opinions have usually been deleted. In some cases minor changes in spelling and punctuation have been made to improve readibility of the opinions.

---

[3]Most areas covered in this book are unsettled, and one should note that changes in the legal-medical area frequently differ dramatically from jurisdiction to jurisdiction. A few of the cases reported in this book have been reversed wholly or in part on appeal. Some of the other cases remain in the appellate process.

CONTENTS

COURTS AND
MODERN MEDICINE

CHAPTER 1

ABORTION

INTRODUCTION

ONE of the most controversial decisions of the Supreme Court
in the 1970s was *Roe v. Wade*.[1] *Roe* struck down a Texas law
that outlawed all abortions except those to save the life of the woman. In doing so, the Court built upon a body of law which emphasized a right to privacy over reproductive decisions. Such a right,
though not specifically mentioned in the Constitution, was found to
be implied. Thus, the right might be found to be part of "liberty"
protected by the due process clause of the fifth and fourteenth ad-
mendments. It may also be found in the ninth amendment, which
states that rights unmentioned in the Bill of Rights may still be reserved to the states or to the people. Finally, such a right may be
found in the penumbras of the Bill of Rights. That is, since many
rights in the Bill of Rights are designed to protect privacy, the sum of
those rights clearly implies a recognition that reproductive privacy is
fundamental and should be protected.[2]

A basic problem with *Roe*, however, is that the right of reproductive privacy, and certainly the fundamental right to an abortion, is
not specifically found in the Constitution. Justice Burger, for example, has written that the right to privacy has tenuous moorings to the
Constitution, implying that there is a highly subjective element in
the judicial discovery of such a right.[3] The subjective nature of this
right has left the Court open to attack on the ground that it used judicial interpretation to make a major policy decision, one more appropriately left to the political branches of government. Opponents
of the decision have argued that the Constitution must mention
rights before a Court holds that they are fundamental. At least a fundamental right should be one that is deeply engrained in the consciousness of the American people. Opponents of the abortion

---

[1] 410 U.S. 113 (1973).
[2] The best treatment of the sources of the right to privacy is *Griswold v. Connecticut*, 381 U.S. 479 (1965).
[3] See *Eisenstadt v. Baird*, 405 U.S. 438 (1972).

decision argue that abortion hardly meets that standard.[4]

ABORTION AND PRIVACY IN THE PAST

Nevertheless, one can find support for the Court's decision in both the common law and in precedent. Under the common law, abortion prior to quickening was not considered a crime. Quickening was the point at which there was noticeable fetal movement. Though such a point varies from one pregnancy to another, quickening generally would occur late in the fourth or early in the fifth month of pregnancy. Abortion of a quickened fetus was considered a crime. Early in the 1800s, England made prequickened abortions a crime. America did not rapidly follow England's lead. In 1850, only seventeen states had abortion laws. During the period 1840-1880, the incidence of abortion in the United States was very high. Estimates are that for every five to six births during this period, there was one abortion.[5]

It was not until the period from 1880-1900 that the United States ended its tolerance for abortion and officially proscribed it. That change was due to religious activity in opposition to abortion, the political efforts of those who saw abortion as a threat to the nation's sexual morality, and the increasing professionalism of medicine and control over medical practices by doctors. As a result, efforts by the states to restrict early abortions are relatively new.[6]

There was also a considerable body of precedent that supported the Court's decision in *Roe v. Wade*. For example, in *Skinner v. Okla-*

---

[4]See the dissenting opinion in *Roe v. Wade*, op cit. While public opinion is usually too much in flux to be useful in determing whether a right is fundamental, it is nevertheless useful to note public attitudes toward abortion. Polls on abortion conducted from 1965-1980 by the National Opinion Research Center asked people whether abortion "should be possible for a pregnant woman to obtain: (1) if the woman's health is seriously endangered by the pregnancy; (2) if she became pregnant as a result of rape; (3) if there is a strong chance of a serious defect in the baby; (4) if the family has a very low income and cannot afford any more children; (5) if she is not married and does not want to marry the man; (6) if she is married and does not want any more children." Over the years there has been a pattern of increased support for abortion for all reasons with the increase in pro abortion views especially great in 1974, the year after *Roe v. Wade*. By 1974, from 85 percent to 92 percent approved of abortion for the first three reasons and from 47 percent to 55 percent approved for the last three reasons. Polenberg, Richard: The second victory of Anthony Comstock? (*Society, 19*:37-38, 1982).
[5]Mohr, James C.:*Abortion in America* (New York, Oxford University Press, 1978, pp.20-85).
[6]Ibid.,pp. 200-245.

homa[7] the Court suggested that there was a fundamental right of reproductive privacy. Though the Court's reasoning was *dicta*, not essential to the decision of the Court, it was said that Oklahoma could not sterilize an habitual thief since such a practice would interfere with the thief's fundamental right to reproduce. In *Griswold v. Connecticut*,[8] the Court struck down a statute that forbade married people from using birth control. Such a law, argued the Court, was an interference with marital privacy and beyond the power of the state. Shortly before the *Roe* decision, the Court decided *Eisenstadt v. Baird*.[9] There, the Court struck down a law forbidding the use of birth control by unmarried persons. Again, the justification for the Court's action was based on reproductive privacy. While such precedents did not compel the Court to decide *Roe* as it did, the Court's reasoning in these earlier decisions provides support for the Court's reasoning in *Roe*.

It must also be recognized that judges are products of the political and social environment and are affected by that environment. *Roe* came after a twenty-year period of judicial activism in the civil liberties areas which was unsurpassed in American history. Judges had, during this period, become accustomed to making policy decisions, especially when those decisions could be framed in concepts of fundamental rights and individual liberty.[10] The women's rights movement had become a powerful force in American society. The Court in this period had proven quite responsive to the interests of women, and abortion was a women's rights issue.[11] Social values were increasingly tolerant of abortion. Some states, such as New York, California, Hawaii, Colorado, and Washington, had passed laws that allowed early-term abortions.[12] There had been considerable publicity surrounding the danger and expense of illegal abortions, and women were still undergoing abortions in spite of the restrictive abortion laws. Often, however, they were paying exorbitant prices to illegal abortionists, who often performed abortions in

---

[7]316 U.S. 535 (1942).

[8]381 U.S. 479 (1965).

[9]405 U.S. 438 (1972).

[10]Horowitz, Donald L.: *The Courts and Social Policy* (Washington, D.C., The Brookings Institute, 1977).

[11]Goldstein, Leslie Friedman: *The Constitutional Rights of Women* (New York, Longman, 1979, pp. 95-98, 271-275).

[12]Granberg, Donald; and Denney, Donald: The coathanger and the rose (*Society, 19*:39, 1982).

an unsafe manner. Yet, medical technology was such that abortion should have been a quick, safe, and inexpensive procedure, especially when the abortion was performed in the early stages of pregnancy.

The justices must have also been aware of and been affected by the tragic stories surrounding both the thalidomide tragedy and the rubella epidemic in the early 1960s. Both events had led to the births of terribly deformed infants; both also led to well-publicized efforts of women to obtain abortions in order to avoid the births of such infants. Sympathy for these women and support for abortion was aroused by their plight of being forced to give birth in such circumstances.[13]

THE COURT'S REASONING

Such was the environment of the *Roe* decision. The Court struck down an old abortion law, one passed in the late nineteenth century. It was an extremely restrictive law, one which limited abortions to those necessary to save the life of the woman. In striking down the Texas law, however, the Court made it clear that the right to an abortion was not absolute. Instead, that right had to be balanced against legitimate state interests in restricting abortions. Those state interests included protecting the health of the woman and protecting fetal life. The interests were balanced in such a way that in the first trimester of pregnancy the decision to abort was to be made by the woman in consultation with her physician. At this point the privacy interests of the woman were considered especially great since state interests were minimal. The state could not argue that abortion must be forbidden in order to protect the health of the woman since first-trimester abortions are very safe. Nor was the state's interest in protecting fetal life great since the fetus was not viable at this point. The Court noted that one could not argue that the nonviable fetus was a constitutionally protected person since the constitutional concept of personhood was postnatal. The second trimester of pregnancy allowed the state greater regulatory powers over abortion since second-trimester abortions were more dangerous to the health of the woman. In the third trimester the state's interests outweighed

---

[13]Mohr, op cit., pp. 252-253.

the privacy interests of the woman. Not only was there considerably more danger to the health of the woman in the third trimester, but the state's interest in protecting fetal life was now quite strong since in this trimester the fetus was viable.

POST-*ROE* ATTEMPTS TO RESTRICT ABORTIONS

With *Roe* and its companion case, *Doe v. Bolton*,[14] both nineteenth century and modern statutes were struck down as violating a woman's right to privacy. The next step was to determine which state regulations limited unconstitutionally the right to an abortion. Such restrictive laws continue to be passed by state legislatures and local governments. Efforts to limit the impact of *Roe* have not been limited to legislative efforts to limit access to abortion. There have also been widespread attempts to picket abortion clinics and in some cases these efforts have been violent. Attempts have also been made to amend the Constitution in order to reverse *Roe v. Wade*. These proposed amendments include a state's rights amendment. The amendment has had various forms but all reflect the thinking of the version introduced in 1975. This amendment states, "The Congress within Federal jurisdiction and the several states within their jurisdictions shall have power to protect life including the unborn at every stage of biological development irrespective of age, health, or condition of physical dependency."[15] A second amendment, often called the "human life amendment" was first introduced in Congress in 1977. The amendment states:

> Section 1. With respect to the right to life the word person, as used in this article and in the fifth and fourteenth articles of amendment to the Constitution of the United States, applies to all human beings, irrespective of age, health, function, or condition of dependency, including their unborn offspring at every stage of their biological development. Section 2. No unborn person shall be deprived of life by any person: provided, however, that nothing in this article shall prohibit a law permitting only those medical procedures required to prevent the death of the mother. Section 3. Congress and the several States shall have the power to enforce this article by appropriate legislation within their respective jurisdictions.[16]

---

[14]410 U.S. 179 (1973).
[15]Rice, Charles E.:*Beyond Abortion* (Chicago, Franciscan Herald Press, 1979, p. 107).
[16]Ibid., pp. 108-109.

The most prohibitive amendment, commonly known as the Helms amendment for its sponsor Senator Jesse Helms, was also introduced in Congress for the first time in 1977. The Helms amendment states: "Section 1. With respect to the right to life guaranteed in this Constitution, every human being, subject to the jurisdiction of the United States, or of any State, shall be deemed, from the moment of fertilization, to be a person and entitled to the right to life. Section 2.Congress and the several States shall have concurrent power to enforce this article by appropriate legislation."[17]

One problem faced by the antiabortion forces is that the existence of three major amendments divide those forces. That division is essentially focused on the basis of commitment to the principle that there should be no abortion. The state's rights amendment, for example, reverses *Roe* and returns the abortion controversy to the pre-*Roe* situation of allowing the political process to determine whether fetal life should be protected. The strongest opponents of abortion, however, oppose the amendment on the grounds that it would allow a state to legislate in favor of abortion. The human rights amendment has stronger support among pro-life forces, but it is also far more restrictive than the state's rights amendment. The amendment has been criticized for a lack of clarity in defining the beginning of constitutional protections. It is unclear when one is an "offspring." Dedicated pro-life advocates prefer a clear definition that constitutional protections begin at the moment of fertilization. There is also some concern that Section 2 of the amendment provides too great an exception to the ban on abortions. In particular, there is a fear that abortions would be legal under a psychiatric justification, such that the threat of suicide would allow abortion. There is also a problem that Section 2 is so poorly worded that it appears a constitutional violation would occur if an accident led to miscarriage. The Helms amendment is by far the most restrictive of the antiabortion amendments. Its language appears to ban some forms of birth control. There is also no language in the amendment for allowing an abortion if the woman's life is endangered, although one may argue that such an exception is implied but not specific to prevent the possibility of easy psychiatric abortions. Interestingly, neither the human

---

[17]Ibid., pp. 110.

life amendment nor the Helms amendment would allow non-life-endangering abortions where pregnancy is the result of rape or incest. With the state's rights anti-abortion amendment, each state would decide whether or not to allow abortions for pregnancy resulting from rape or incest.[18]

The amendments have considerable support, but it is extremely difficult to pass a constitutional amendment, so difficult that the passage of any amendment is unlikely. Congress must propose an amendment by a two-thirds vote of each house and the legislatures of three-fourths of the states must ratify it. Another amendment method, which is probably more cumbersome, would require two-thirds of the states to petition Congress to call a constitutional convention. The convention would then propose amendments that would have to be ratified by three-fourths of the states.

Recognizing the difficulty of amending the Constitution, anti-abortion forces are attempting two other efforts that could reverse *Roe*. An attempt is being made to remove abortion cases from the jurisdiction of federal courts. Since most of the jurisdiction of federal courts is determined by statute, antiabortion forces argue that only a Congressional statute is needed to remove abortion from federal court jurisdiction. If there were no recourse to the federal courts, it might be possible to legislate restrictions on abortions and prevent proabortion forces from obtaining judicial recourse. The other effort to reverse *Roe* involves the definition of a person. The human life statute provides that "actual human life exists from conception."[19] Thus, the unborn would be considered a legal person and would be protected by the Constitution. Such a statute could be passed by a simple majority of Congress. It is argued that the effect of the statute would be to reverse *Roe*. *Roe* held that the constitutional concept of "person" applied postnatally, but this expanded definition would create prenatal persons as well.

Another method of restricting access to abortion involves the refusal of states and the national government to provide funds for

---

[18]Ibid., pp. 108-111.

[19]Davis, Jessica G.: Legislating science. (*Society*, *19*:63-64, 1982); Milansky, Aubrey; and Glantz, Leonard H.: Abortion legislation (*The Journal of the American Medical Association*, *248*:833-834, 1982); Press, Aric; Comper, Diane; and Lindsay, John L.: "Congress's Court Stingyness" (*Newsweek*, *97*:67, 1982).

abortions for poor women. In *Maher v. Roe*,[20] the Supreme Court upheld Connecticut's refusal to provide state funds for abortions except where those abortions were medically necessary. The more restrictive Hyde amendment prohibited the use of federal funds for abortion unless the woman's life was in danger. In both *Maher v. Roe* and the Hyde amendment case, *Harris v. McRae*,[21] the Supreme Court upheld the refusal to provide funds on the grounds that refusal to fund abortions is not a barrier to the exercise of the fundamental right to abortion. The government is free to make a value judgment and fund childbirth while refusing to fund abortion. The real barrier to abortion is not the refusal to fund, but the woman's poverty. Government, however, is under no legal obligation to redress inequities of wealth.

Prior to the Hyde amendment, the federal government was paying for about 295,000 Medicaid abortions a year. Roughly, one-quarter of all abortions in the nation were paid for by Medicaid. In the two years following the Hyde amendment, the federal government paid for an average of about 2,500 abortions a year.[22] Several states continue to pay for abortions for poor women. However, even in states that do not fund abortions, most poor women continue to receive abortions, although they obtain their abortions an average of two weeks later than nonindigent women in those states that continue to fund abortions. Roughly 80 percent of poor women who desire abortions appear to receive abortions without Medicaid funding, but it is likely that they undergo considerable hardships to do so. A study in Ohio, for example, found that indigent women who did not receive Medicaid paid close to the full cost of abortions.[23] A study of twenty-four institutions in fourteen states and the District of Columbia found no significant relationship between the proportion of poor women who had abortion complications in states that fund abortions versus states that do not fund abortions. How-

---

[20]432 U.S. 464 (1977).
[21]448 U.S. 297 (1980).
[22]Segers, Mary C.: Governing abortion policy. In Gambitta, Richard A.L.; May, Marilyn L.; and Foster, James C. (Eds.): *Governing Through Courts* (Beverly Hills, California, Sage Publications, 1981, pp. 290-293).
[23]Ibid; Trussell, James; Menken, Jane; Lindheim, Barbara L.; and Vaughan, Barbara: The impact of restricting medicaid financing for abortion (*Family Planning Perspectives, 12*:120-130, 1980).

ever poor women in states that do not fund abortions had a mean 1.9 week later gestational age at the time of abortion than poor women in states that do not fund abortions. Additionally, in the nonfunding states, poor women had a mean 2.4 week later gestational age than nonpoor women in those states.[24]

TABLE I

Death Rates for Legal Abortions in
the United States (1972-1977)

Weeks of Gestation	Rate of Death per 100,000 abortions
<8	0.6
9-10	1.7
11-12	2.7
13-15	7.5
16-20	14.6
>21	20.5
overall	2.6

Source: Center for Disease Control: Abortion-related mortality—United States, 1977 (*Morbidity and Mortality Weekly, 28*:302, 1979).

THE SAFETY OF LEGAL ABORTION

Legal abortions are quite safe. With well over 1,000,000 legal abortions occurring annually, there has been an average of 21 deaths per year of women which were attributed to abortion between 1972-1977.[25] Table I provides death rates per 100,000 legal abortions according to the weeks of gestation.

[24]Cates, Willard, Jr.; Kimball, Ann Marie; Gold, Julian; Rubin, George L.; Smith, Jack C.; Rochat, Roger W.; and Tyler, Carl W.; Jr.: The health impact of restricting public funds for abortion, October 10, 1977—June 10, 1978 (*American Journal of Public Health, 69*:946, 1979). [25]Center for Disease Control: Abortion-related mortality (*Morbidity and Mortality Weekly Report, 28*:303, 1979). The safety of abortions has recently been stressed. See Cates, Willard, Jr.; Schulz, Kenneth F.; Grimes, David A.; Horowitz, Arthur, J.; Lyon, Fred A.; Kravitz, Fred H.; and Frisch, Melvin J.: Dilatation and evacuation procedures and second-trimester abortions (*The Journal of the American Medical Association, 248*:559-563, 1982); Lebolt, Scott A.; Grimes, David A.; and Cates, Willard, Jr.: Mortality from abortion and childbirth: Are the →

The table suggests that the abortion-related deaths among poor women will increase slightly as a result of the Hyde amendment since lack of Medicaid funding appears to delay the abortion decision by poor women. As the table points out, even a two-week delay in seeking an abortion can increase the chances of the woman's death.

If one divides these data into trimesters, one can see the reasoning behind the trimester division in *Roe v. Wade*. Abortions in the first trimester of pregnancy have an extremely low death rate for women. After the first trimester, however, the death rate significantly increases so that abortions performed at the end of the second trimester have a death rate for women that is thirty-four times the rate in the earliest months of pregnancy.

Table II provides death rates for legal abortions by procedure. Curettage is by far the safest abortion procedure, followed by dilatation and evacuation. Instillation procedures are somewhat more dangerous. As would be expected, the most dangerous procedures are hysterotomy and hysterectomy. One should note that the effort to restrict saline instillation might require hysterotomy or hysterectomy if prostaglandin were unavailable. Yet such procedures are roughly three times more likely to result in the death of the woman than saline instillation. If prostaglandin were available, the table suggests that it would be safer than saline instillation. Since the abortion procedure used is largely a function of the length of gestation, Table II again stresses that the risk to the woman's life increases as delay in seeking an abortion increases.

populations comparable? (*The Journal of the American Medical Association, 248*:188-191, 1982); Cates, Willard, Jr.; Smith, Jack C.; Rochat, Roger W.; and Grimes, David A.: Mortality from abortion and childbirth: Are the statistics biased? (*The Journal of the American Medical Association, 248*:192-196, 1982). Lebolt et al., argue that the death rate for women in childbirth is seven times the death rate for women undergoing abortions.

TABLE II

DEATH RATES by ABORTION PROCEDURE
(1972-1977)

Type of Procedure	Death Rate per 100,000 Abortions
Currettage	1.2
Dilatation and Evacuation	8.3
Prostglandin Instillation*	10.8
Saline Instillation	15.5
Hysterotomy/Hysterectomy	45.3
Overall	2.6

*Includes instillation of other agents.

Source:Center for Disease Control. Abortion-related mortality — United States, 1977 (*Morbidity and Mortality Weekly, 28*:302, 1979).

ROE V. WADE

(U.S. Supreme Court, 1973)
410 U.S. 113

Jane Roe, an unmarried, pregnant female sought a declaratory judgment that the Texas criminal abortion statutes were unconstitutionally vague and that they abridged her right to personal privacy.

MR. JUSTICE BLACKMUN FOR THE COURT:

* * *

"...[W]e accept as true, and as established, her existence; her pregnant state, as of the inception of her suit in March 1970....

* * *

"The usual rule in federal cases is that an actual controversy must exist at stages of appellate or certiorari review, and not simply at the date the action is initiated....

"...[W]hen, as here, pregnancy is a significant fact in the litigation, the normal 266-day human gestation period is so short that the pregnancy will come to term before the usual appellate process is complete. If that termination makes a case moot, pregnancy litigation seldom will survive much beyond the trial stage, and appellate review will be effectively denied. Our law should not be that rigid....

* * *

"The principal thrust of appellant's attack on the Texas statutes is that they improperly invade a right, said to be possessed by the pregnant woman, to choose to terminate her pregnancy. Appellant would discover this right in the concept of personal 'liberty' embodied in the Fourteenth Amendment's Due Process Clause; or in personal, marital, familial, and sexual privacy said to be protected by the Bill of Rights or its penumbras....

"It perhaps is not generally appreciated that the restrictive criminal abortion laws in effect in a majority of States today are of relatively recent vintage. Those laws, generally proscribing abortion or its attempt at any time during pregnancy except when necessary to preserve the pregnant woman's life, are not of ancient or even of common-law origin. Instead, they derive from statutory changes effected, for the most part, in the latter half of the nineteenth century.

***

"Three reasons have been advanced to explain historically the enactment of criminal abortion laws in the nineteenth century and to justify their continued existence.

"It has been argued occasionally that these laws were the product of a Victorian social concern to discourage illicit sexual conduct. Texas, however, does not advance this justification in the present case, and it appears that no court or commentator has taken the argument seriously....

"A second reason is concerned with abortion as a medical procedure. When most criminal abortion laws were first enacted, the procedure was a hazardous one for the woman.... Thus, it has been argued that a State's real concern in enacting a criminal abortion law was to protect the pregnant women, that is, to restrain her from submitting to a procedure that placed her life in serious jeopardy.

"Modern medical techniques have altered this situation. Appellants and various *amici* refer to medical data indicating that abortion in early pregnancy, that is, prior to the end of the first trimester, although not without its risk, is now relatively safe. Mortality rates for women undergoing early abortions, where the procedure is legal, appear to be as low as or lower than the rates for normal childbirth. Consequently, any interest of the State in protecting the woman from an inherently hazardous procedure...has largely disappeared.... The State has a legitimate interest in seeing to it that abortion, like any other medical procedure, is performed under circumstances that insure maximum safety for the patient....

"The third reason is the State's interest — some phrase it in terms of duty — in protecting prenatal life.... In assessing the State's interest, recognition may be given to the less rigid claim that as long as at least *potential* life is involved, the state may assert interests beyond the protection of the pregnant women alone.

* * *

"It is with these interests, and the weight to be attached to them, that this case is concerned.

"The Constitution does not explicitly mention any right of privacy. In a line of decisions, however, going back perhaps as far as *Union Pacific R. Co, v. Botsford*...(1891), the Court has recognized that a right of personal privacy, or a guarantee of certain areas or zones of privacy, does exist under the Constitution. In varying contexts, the Court or individual Justices have, indeed, found at least the roots of that right in the First Amendment, *Stanley v. Georgia*..., in the Fourth and Fifth Amendments, *Terry v. Ohio*..., *Katz v. United States*..., in the penumbras of the Bill of Rights, *Griswold v. Connecticut*..., in the Ninth Amendment, *id.*, (Goldberg, J., concurring); or in the concept of liberty guaranteed by the first section of the Fourteenth Amendment, see *Meyer v. Nebraska*.... These decisions make it clear that only personal rights that can be deemed "fundamental" or "Implicit in the concept of ordered liberty," *Palko v. Connecticut*..., are included in this guarantee of personal privacy. They also make it clear that the right has some extension to activities relating to marriage, *Loving v. Virginia*...; procreation, *Skinner v. Oklahoma*...; contraception, *Eisenstadt v. Baird*...; family relationships, *Prince v. Massachusetts*...; and child rearing and education, *Pierce v. Society of Sisters*....

"This right of privacy, whether it be founded in the Fourteenth Amendment's concept of personal liberty and restrictions upon state action, as we feel it is, or, as the District Court determined, in the Ninth Amendment's reservation of rights to the people, is broad enough to encompass a women's decision whether or not to terminate her pregnancy. The detriment that the State would impose upon the pregnant women by denying this choice altogether is apparent. Specific and direct harm medically diagnosable even in early pregnancy may be involved. Maternity, or additional offspring, may force upon the woman a distressful life and future. Psychological harm may be imminent. Mental and physical health may be taxed by child care. There is also the distress, for all concerned, associated with the unwanted child, there is the problem of bringing a child into a family already unable, psychologically and otherwise, to care for it. In other cases, as in this one, the additional difficulties and continuing stigma of unwed motherhood may be involved. All these are factors the woman and her responsible physician necessarily will consider in consultation.

"On the basis of elements such as these, appellant and some *amici* argue that the woman's right is absolute and that she is entitled to terminate her pregnancy at whatever time, in whatever way, and for whatever reason she alone chooses. With this we do not agree....

"We...conclude that the right of personal privacy includes the abortion decision, but that this right is not unqualified and must be considered against important state interests in regulation.

* * *

"Where certain 'fundamental rights' are involved, the Court has held that regulation limiting these rights may be justified only by a "compelling state interest"...and that legislative enactments must be narrowly drawn to express only the legitimate state interests at stake....

* * *

"The appellee and certain *amici* argue that the fetus is a 'person' within the language and meaning of the Fourteenth Amendment. In support of this, they outline at length and in detail the well-known facts of fetal development. If this suggestion of personhood is established, the appellant's case, of course, collapses, for the fetus' right to life would then be guaranteed specifically by the Amendment....

"The Constitution does not define 'person' in so many words. Section 1 of the Fourteenth Amendment contains three references to 'person.' The first, in defining 'citizens,' speaks of 'persons born or naturalized in the United States.' The word also appears both in the Due Process Clause and in the Equal Protection Clause. 'Person' is used in other places in the Constitution: in the listing of qualifications for Representatives and Senators,...in the Apportionment Clause,...in the Migration and Importation provision,...in the Emolument Clause,...in the Electors provisions,...and the superseded cl.3; in the provision outlining qualifications for the office of President,...in the Extradition provisions,...and the superseded Fugitive Slave Clause,...and in the Fifth, Twelfth, and Twenty-second Amendments, as well as in §2 and 3 of the Fourteenth Amendment. But in nearly all these instances, the use of the word is such that it has application only postnatally. None indicates with any assurance that it has any possible prenatal application.

"All this, together with our observation, *supra*, that throughout the major portion of the nineteenth century prevailing legal abortion practices were far freer than they are today, persuades us that the word 'person,' as used in the Fourteenth Amendment, does not include the unborn....

"This conclusion, however, does not of itself fully answer the contentions raised by Texas, and we pass on to other considerations.

"The pregnant woman cannot be isolated in her privacy. She carries an embryo and, later, a fetus, if one accepts the medical definitions of the developing young in the human uterus.... This situation therefore is inherently different from marital intimacy, or bedroom possession of obscene material, or marriage, or procreation, or education, with which *Eisenstadt* and *Griswold, Stanley, Loving, Skinner* and *Pierce* and *Meyer* were respectively concerned....

"Texas urges that, apart from the Fourteenth Amendment, life begins at conception and is present throughout pregnancy, and that, therefore, the State has a compelling interest in protecting that life from and after conception. We need not resolve the difficult question of when life begins. When those trained in the respective disciplines of medicine, philosophy, and theology are unable to arrive at any consensus, the judiciary, at this point in the development of man's knowledge, is not in a position to speculate as to the answer.

* * *

"[W]e do not agree that, by adopting one theory of life, Texas may override the rights of the pregnant women that are at stake. We repeat, however, that the state does have an important and legitimate interest in preserving and protecting the health of the pregnant woman, whether she be a resident of the State or a non-resident who seeks medical consultation and treatment there, and that it has still *another* important and legitimate interest in protecting the potentiality of human life. These interests are separate and distinct. Each grows in substantiality as the woman approaches term and, at a point during pregnancy, each becomes 'compelling.'

"With respect to the State's important and legitimate interest in the health of the mother, the 'compelling' point, in the light of present medical knowledge, is at approximately the end of the first trimester. This is so because of the now-established medical fact, referred to above, that until the end of the first trimester, mortality in abortion may be less than mortality in normal childbirth. It follows that from and after this point, a State may regulate the abortion procedure to the extent that the regulation reasonably relates to the preservation and protection of maternal health. Examples of permissible state regulation in this area are requirements as to the qualifications of the person who is to perform the abortion; as to the licensure of that person; as to the facility in which the procedure is to be performed, that is, whether it must be a hospital or may be a clinic or some other place of less-than-hospital status; as to the licensing of the facility; and the like.

"This means, on the other hand, that, for the period prior to this 'compelling' point, the attending physician, in consultation with his patient, is free to determine, without regulation by the State, that, in his medical judgment, the patient's pregnancy should be terminated. If that decision is reached, the judgment may be effectuated by an abortion free of interference by the State.

"With respect to the state's important and legitimate interest in potential life, the 'compelling' point is at viability. This is so because the fetus then presumably has the capability of meaningful life outside the mother's womb. State regulation protective of fetal life after viability thus has both logical and biological justifications. If the State is interested in protecting fetal life after viability, it may go so far as to proscribe abortion during that period, except when it is necessary to preserve the life or health of the mother.

"Measured against these standards, Art. 1196 of the Texas Penal Code...sweeps too broadly. The statute makes no distinction between abortions performed early in pregnancy and those performed later, and it limits to a single reason, 'saving' the mother's life, the legal justification for the procedure. The statute, therefore, cannot survive the constitutional attack made upon it here."

* * *

JUSTICE REHNQUIST DISSENTING:

* * *

"...I have difficulty in concluding, as the Court does, that the right of 'privacy' is involved in this case. Texas, by the statute here challenged, bars the performance of a medical abortion by a licensed physician on a plaintiff such as Roe. A transaction resulting in an operation such as this is not 'private' in the ordinary usage of that word. Nor is the 'privacy' that the Court finds here even a distant relative of the freedom from searches and seizures protected by the Fourth Amendment to the Constitution, which the Court has referred to as embodying a right to privacy....

"If the Court means by the term 'privacy' no more than that the claim of a person to be free from unwanted state regulation of consensual transactions may be a form of 'liberty' protected by the Fourteenth Amendment, there is no doubt that similar claims have been upheld in our earlier decisions on the basis of that liberty. I agree with the statement of Mr. Justice Stewart in his concurring opinion that the 'liberty', against deprivation of which without due process the Fourteenth Amendment protects, embraces more than the rights found in the Bill of Rights. But that liberty is not guaranteed absolutely against deprivation, only against deprivation without due process of law. The test traditionally applied in the area of social and economic legislation is whether or not a law such as that challenged has a rational relation to a valid state objective... If the Texas statute were to prohibit an abortion even where the mother's life is in jeopardy, I have little doubt that such a statue would lack a rational relation to a valid state objective.... But the Court's sweeping invalidation of any restriction is impossible to justify under that standard and the conscious weighing of competing factors that the Court's opinion apparently substitutes for the established test is far more appropriate to a legislative judgment than to a judicial one.

***

"...The decision here to break pregnancy into three distinct terms and to outline the permissible restrictions the State may impose in each one, for example, partakes more of judicial legislation than it does of a determination of the intent of the drafters of the Fourteenth Amendment.

"The fact that a majority of the states reflecting, after all the majority sentiment in those States, have had restrictions on abortions for at least a century is a strong indication, it seems to me, that the asserted right to an abortion is not 'so rooted in the traditions and conscience of our people as to be ranked as fundamental....' Even today, when society's views on abortion are changing, the very existence of the debate is evidence that the 'right' to an abortion is not so universally accepted as the appellant would have us believe. To reach its result, the Court necessarily has had to find within the Scope of the Fourteenth Amendment a right that was apparently completely unknown to the drafters of the Amendment. As early as 1821, the first state law dealing directly with abortion was enacted by the Connecticut Legislature.... By the time of the adoption of the Fourteenth Amendment in 1868, there were at least 36 laws enacted by state or territorial legislatures limiting abortion. While many States have amended or updated their laws, 21 of the laws on the books in 1868 remain in effect today. Indeed, the Texas statute struck down today was, as the majority notes, first enacted in 1857 and 'has remained substantially unchanged to the present time....'

"There apparently was no question concerning the validity of this provision or of any of the other states statutes when the Fourteenth Amendment was adopted. The only conclusions possible from this history is that the drafters did not intend to have the Fourteenth Amendment withdraw from the states the power to legislate with respect to this matter."

***

(Concurring opinions by Chief Justice Burger, Justice Stewart, and Justice Douglas are deleted. A dissenting opinion by Justice White is also deleted.)

PLANNED PARENTHOOD
OF CENTRAL MISSOURI V. DANFORTH

(U.S. Supreme Court, 1976)
428 U.S. 52

What are some of the ways that are and are not permissible regulations of abortion?

JUSTICE BLACKMUN DELIVERED THE OPINION OF THE COURT:

"This case is a logical and anticipated corollary to *Roe v. Wade*...and *Doe v. Bolton*...for it raises issues secondary to those that were then before the Court. Indeed, some of the questions now presented were forecast and reserved in *Roe* and *Doe*...

"The definition of viability, Section 2(2) of the Act defines 'viability' as 'that stage of fetal development when the life of the unborn child may be continued indefinitely outside the womb by natural or artificial life-support systems.' Appellants claim that this definition to contain any reference to a gestational time period, to its failure to incorporate and reflect the three stages of pregnancy, to the presence of the word 'indefinitely,' and to the extra burden of failure to incorporate and reflect the three stages of pregnancy, to the presence of the word 'indefinitely,' and to be extra burden of regulation imposed. It is suggested that the definition expands the Court's definition of viability, as expressed in *Roe*, and amounts to a legislative determination of what is properly a matter for medical judgment. It is said that the 'mere possibility of momentary survival is not the medical standard of viability....'

"In *Roe*, we used the term 'viable,' properly we thought, to signify the point at which the fetus is 'potentially able to live outside the mother's womb, albeit with artificial aid,' and presumably capable of 'meaningful life outside the mother's womb....' We noted that this point 'is usually placed' at about seven months or 28 weeks, but may occur ealier....

"We agree with the District Court and conclude that the definition of viability in the Act does not conflict with what was said and held in *Roe*. In fact, we believe that section 2(2), even when read in conjunction with section 5 (proscribing an abortion 'not necessary to preserve the life or health of the mother—unless the attending physician first certifies with reasonable medical certainty that the fetus is not viable'), the constitutionality of which is not explicitly challenged here, reflects an attempt on the part of the Missouri General Assembly to comply with our observations and discussion in *Roe* relating to viability....

"In any event, we agree with the District Court that it is not the proper function of the legislature or the courts to place viability, which essentially is a medical concept, at a specific point in the gestation period. The time when viability is achieved may vary with each pregnancy, and the determination of whether a particular fetus is viable is, and must be, a matter for the judgment of the responsible attending physician. The definition of viability in section 2(2) merely reflects this fact. The appellees do not contend otherwise, for they insist that the determination of viability rests with the physician in the exercise of his professional judgment.

We thus do not accept appellants' contention that a specified number of weeks in pregnancy must be fixed by statute as the point of viability....

***

"THE WOMAN'S CONSENT. Under section 3(2) of the Act, a woman prior to submitting to an abortion during the first 12 weeks of pregnancy, must certify in writing her consent to the procedure and 'that her consent is informed and freely given and is not the result of coercion.' Appellants argue that this requirement is violative of *Roe v. Wade*...by imposing an extra layer and burden of regulation on the abortion decision.... Appellants also claim that the provision is overboard and vague.

"The District Court's majority relied on the propositions that the decision to terminate a pregnancy, of course, 'is often a stressful one,' and that the consent requirement of section 3(2) 'insures that the pregnant woman retains control over the discretions of her consulting physician....' The majority also felt that the consent requirement 'does not single out the abortion procedure, but merely includes it within the category of medical operations for which consent is required....'

"We do not disagree with the result reached by the District Court as to section 3(2). It is true that *Doe* and *Roe* clearly establish the State may not restrict the decision of the patient and her physician regarding abortion during the first stage of pregnancy.... [T]he imposition by section 3(2) of such a requirement for termination of pregnancy even during the first stage, in our view, is not in itself an unconstitutional requirement. The decision to abort, indeed, is an important and often a stressful one, and it is desirable and imperative that it be made with full knowledge of its nature and consequences. The woman is the one primarily concerned, and her awareness of the decision and its significance may be assured, constitutionally, by the State to the extent of requiring her prior written consent.

* * *

"THE SPOUSE'S CONSENT. Section 3(3) requires the prior written consent of the spouse of the woman seeking an abortion during the first 12 weeks of pregnancy, unless 'the abortion is certified by a licensed physician to be necessary in order to preserve the life of the mother.'

"The appellees defend section 3(3) on the ground that it was enacted in the light of the General Assembly's 'perception of marriage as an institution,'...and that any major change in family status is a decision to be made jointly by the marriage partners....

* * *

"We now hold that the State may not constitutionally require the consent of the spouse, as is specified under section 3(3) of the Missouri Act, as a condition for abortion during the first 12 weeks of pregnancy. We thus agree with the dissenting judge in the present case,...that the State cannot 'delegate to a spouse a veto power which the state itself is absolutely and totally prohibited from exercising during the first trimester of pregnancy'.... Clearly, since the State cannot regulate or proscribe abortion during the first stage, when the physician and his patient make that decision, the State cannot delegate authority to any particular person, even the spouse, to prevent abortion during the same period.

"We are not unaware of the deep and proper concern and interest that a devoted and protective husband has in his wife's pregnancy and in the growth and development of the fetus she is carrying. Neither has this Court failed to appreciate the importance of the marital relationship in our society.... Moreover, we recognize that the decision whether to undergo or to forego an abortion may have profound effects on the future of any marriage, effects that are both physical and mental, and possibly deleterious. Notwithstanding these factors, we cannot hold that the State has the constitutional authority to give the spouse unilaterally the ability to prohibit the wife from terminating her pregnancy, when the state itself lacks that right....

It seems manifest that, ideally, the decision to terminate a pregnancy should be one concurred in by both the wife and her husband. No marriage may be viewed as harmonious or successful if the marriage partners are fundamentally divided on so important and vital an issue. But it is difficult to believe that the goal of fostering mutuality and trust in a marriage, and of strengthening the marital relationship and the marriage institution, will be achieved by giving the husband a veto power exercisable for any reason whatsoever or for no reason at all. Even if the State had the ability to delegate to the husband a power it itself could not exercise, it is not at all likely that such action would further, as the District Court majority phrased it, the 'interest of the state in protecting the mutuality of decisions vital to the marriage relationship'....

"We recognize, of course, that when a woman, with the approval of her physician but without the approval of her husband, decides to terminate her pregnancy, it could be said that she is acting unilaterally. The obvious fact is that when the wife and the husband disagree on this decision, the view of only one of the two marriage partners can prevail. Inasmuch as it is the woman who physically bears the child and who is the more directly and immediately affected by the pregnancy, as between the two, the balance weighs in her favor....

***

"PARENTAL CONSENT. Section 3(4) requires, with respect to the first 12 weeks of pregnancy, where the woman is unmarried and under the age of 18 years, the written consent of a parent or person *in loco parentis* unless, again, 'the abortion is certified by a licensed physician as necessary in order to preserve the life of the mother.' It is to be observed that only one parent need consent.

***

"Constitutional rights do not mature and come into being magically only when one attains the state-defined age of majority. Minors, as well as adults, are protected by the Constitution and possess constitutional rights.... The Court indeed, however, long has recognized that the State has somewhat broader authority to regulate the activities of children than of adults.... It remains, then, to examine whether there is any significant state interest in conditioning an abortion on the consent of a parent or person *in loco parentis* that is not present in the case of an adult.

"One suggested interest is the safeguarding of the family unit and of parental authority.... It is difficult, however, to conclude that providing a parent with absolute power to overrule a determination, made by the physician and his minor patient, to terminate the patient's pregnancy will serve to strengthen the family unit. Neither is it likely that such veto power will enhance parental authority or control where the minor and the nonconsenting parent are so fundamentally in conflict and the very existence of the pregnancy already has fractured the family structure. An independent interest the parent may have in the termination of the minor daughter's pregnancy is no more weighty than the right of privacy of the competent minor mature enough to have become pregnant.

"We emphasize that our holding that section 3(4) is invalid does not suggest that every minor, regardless of age or maturity, may give effective consent for termination of her pregnancy.... The fault with section 3(4) is that it imposes a special-consent provision, exercisable by a person other than the woman and her physician, as a prerequisite to a minor's termination of her pregnancy and does so without a sufficient justification for the restriction....

"Saline amniocentesis.Section 9 of the statute prohibits the use of saline amniocentesis, as a method or technique of abortion, after the first 12 weeks of pregnancy. It describes the method as one whereby the amniotic fluid is withdrawn and 'a saline or other fluid' is inserted into the amniotic sac. The statute imposes this proscription on the ground that the technique 'is deleterious to maternal health....' Appellants challenge this provision on the ground that it operates to preclude virtually all abortions after the first trimester. This is so, it is claimed, because a substantial percentage, in the neighborhood of 70 percent according to the testimony, of all abortions performed in the United States after the first trimester are effected through the procedure of saline amniocentesis. Appellants stress the fact that the alternative methods of hysterotomy and hysterectomy are significantly more dangerous and critical for the woman than the saline technique; they also point out that the mortality rate for normal childbirth exceeds that where saline amniocentesis is employed. Finally, appellants note that the perhaps safer alternative of prostaglandin instillation, suggested and strongly relied upon by the appellees, at least at the time of the trial, is not yet widely used in this country.

***

"The District Court's majority determined, on the basis of the evidence before it, that the maternal mortality rate in childbirth does, indeed, exceed the mortality rate where saline amniocentesis is used.

Therefore, the majority acknowledged, section 9 could be upheld only if there were safe alternative methods of inducing abortion after the first 12 weeks.... Referring to such methods as hysterotomy, hysterectomy, 'mechanical means of inducing abortion', and prostaglandin injection, the majority said that at least the latter two techniques were safer than saline. Consequently, the majority concluded, the restriction in section 9 could be upheld as reasonably related to maternal health.

"We feel that the majority, in reaching its conclusion, failed to appreciate and to consider several significant facts. First, it did not recognize the prevalence, as the record conclusively demonstrates, of the use of saline amniocentesis as an accepted medical procedure in this country; the procedure, as noted above, is employed in a substantial majority (the testimony from both sides ranges from 68% to 80%) of all post-first-trimester abortions. Second, it failed to recognize that at the time of trial, there were several limitations on the availability of the prostaglandin technique, which, although promising, was used only on an experimental basis until less than two years before.... Third, the statute's reference to the insertion of 'a saline or other fluid' appears to include within its proscription the intraamniotic injection of protaglandin itself and other methods that may be developed in the future and that may prove highly effective and completely safe. Finally, the majority did not consider the anomaly inherent in section 9 when it proscribes the use of saline but does not prohibit techniques that are many times more likely to result in maternal death....

***

"As so viewed, particularly in the light of the present unavailability—as demonstrated by the record—of the prostaglandin technique, the outright legislative proscription of saline fails as a reasonable regulation for the protection of maternal health. It comes into focus, instead, as an unreasonable or arbitrary regulation designed to inhibit, and having the effect of inhibiting, the vast majority of abortions after the first 12 weeks. As such, it does not withstand constitutional challenge....

"RECORDKEEPING. Sections 10 and 11 of the Act impose recordkeeping requirements for health facilities and physicians concerned with abortions irrespective of the pregnancy stage. Under section

10, each such facility and physician is to be supplied with forms 'the purpose and function of which shall be the preservation of maternal health and life by adding to the sum of medical knowledge through the compilation of relevant maternal health and life data and to monitor all abortions performed to assure that they are done only under and in accordance with the provisions of the law.' The statute states that the information on the forms 'shall be confidential and shall be used only for statistical purposes.' The 'records, however, may be inspected and health data acquired by local, state, or national public health officers.' Under section 11 the records are to be kept for seven years in the permanent files of the health facility where the abortion was performed.

* * *

"Recordkeeping and reporting requirements that are reasonably directed to the preservation of maternal health and that properly respect a patient's confidentiality and privacy are permissible.... We conclude...that the provisions of sections 10 and 11, while perhaps approaching impermissible limits, are not constitutionally offensive in themselves. Recordkeeping of this kind, if not abused or overdone, can be useful to the State's interest in protecting the health of its female citizens, and may be a resource that is relevant to decisions involving medical experience and judgment. The added requirements for confidentiality, with the sole exception for public health officers, and for retention for seven years, a period not unreasonable in length, assist and persuade us in our determination of the constitutional limits. As so regarded, we see no legally significant impact or consequence on the abortion decision or on the physician-patient relationship....

"STANDARD OF CARE. Appellee Danforth...appeals from the unanimous decision of the District Court that section 6(1) of the Act is unconstitutional. That section provides: 'No person who performs or induces an abortion shall fail to exercise that degree of professional skill, care and diligence to preserve the life and health of the fetus which such person would be required to exercise in order to preserve the life and health of any fetus intended to be born and not aborted. Any physician or person assisting in the abortion who shall fail to take such measures to encourage or to sustain the life of the child, and the death of the child results, shall be deemed guilty of manslaughter.... Further, such physician or other person shall be liable in an action for damages. The District Court held that the first sentence was unconstitutionally overbroad because it failed to exclude from its reach the stage of pregnancy prior to viability....

* * *

"...Section 6(1) requires the physician to exercise the prescribed skill, care, and diligence to preserve the life and health of the fetus. It does not specify that such care need be taken only after the stage of viability has been reached. As the provision now reads, it impermissibly requires the physician to preserve the life and health of the *fetus*, whatever the stage of the pregnancy. The fact that the second sentence of section 6(1) refers to a criminal penalty where the physician fails 'to take such measures to encourage or to sustain the life of the *child*, and the death of the *child* results'...simply does not modify the duty imposed by the previous sentence or limit the duty to pregnancies that have reached the stage of viability."

* * *

(The concurring opinion of Justice Stewart, joined by Justice Powell, is deleted. The partial concurrence and partial dissent by Justice White, joined by Chief Justice Burger and Justice Rehnquist, is deleted. The partial concurrence and partial dissent of Justice Stevens is also deleted.)

COMMONWEALTH V. EDELIN

(Supreme Judicial Court of Massachusetts, 1976)
359 N.E. 2d 4

Dr. Edelin attempted an abortion by saline injection, but was unable to complete the procedure due to placental placement. Abortion was then done by hysterotomy; a procedure involving an incision of the uterus to manually dislodge the placenta and remove the fetus. The question before the court centered on the hysterotomy procedure in which the placenta was removed prior to checking the viability of the fetus. Does this procedure constitute manslaughter? Initial judgment of guilty was set aside by the appeals court.

JUSTICE KAPLAN:

* * *

"...[A]nalysis of post mortem materials or data led experts for the commonwealth to put the gestational age at the time of the operation at twenty-four weeks, excepting Doctor Ward who went somewhat higher to twenty-six weeks. All recognized that the figures were only estimated. Several prosecution experts would answer in the affirmative the inferential question of 'viability' of the fetus at the time of the operation. The exact import of such judgments turned on the meaning to be ascribed to that term.... In this connection the judge allowed very considerable latitude for the expression by witnesses of medical ideas which he did not relate or channel back to legal standards. For example, the judge did not bring to bear during trial (or, for that matter, in his charge to the jury) the Supreme Court's definition of viability in the relevant sense of the point at which the state might, if it chose, constitutionally assert its interest in bringing the fetus to full term.

* * *

"...The short-form manslaughter indictment, found by the grand jury on April 11, 1974, stated simply 'that [Dr. Edelin] did assault and beat a certain person, to wit: a male child described to the... Jurors as Baby Boy and by such assault and beating did kill the said person.' The Commonwealth was required to respond to an order for particulars of the alleged manslaughter. First, as to when the death of the 'person' has supposedly taken place, the Commonwealth declined the tendered proposition that the death occurred 'when the fetus was totally expelled or removed from the body of the mother,' and adopted the propositions that death occurred 'when Baby Boy with within the mother, and [sic]...when Baby Boy was partially expelled or removed from the body of the mother.' As to the defendant's supposed act claimed to constitute the manslaughter, the Commonwealth particularized that Doctor Edelin's 'act during the course of a hysterotomy, which act constituted manslaughter, was his waiting 3-5 minutes after he manually separated the placenta from the uterine wall and before he removed the person from the abdominal cavity of his mother.'

"From the indictment as particularized, it appeared that the Commonwealth's theory was that, upon the detachment of the placenta, the fetus became a 'person' within the manslaughter statute, and was then killed by a wanton and reckless act of Doctor Edelin, all before the birth of the fetus through its complete delivery clear of the mother's body. The defense asserted by repeated motions that such an accusation would be untenable usage of the manslaughter statute and would, besides, enable the Commonwealth to evade or subvert the constitutional rule of *Wade-Bolton*. The defense contended that manslaughter could be made out, if at all, only where a fetus was born alive completely outside the mother's body and was homicidally destroyed by acts committed at that stage.

"The defense did not persuade the trial judge to limit the case as just indicated and to confine the evidence accordingly....

* * *

"Although the fetus may have been alive in the very narrow sense that there was some postnatal gasping of air as revealed by microscopic analysis of preserved lung tissue long after the event, nothing of the sort was observable by Doctor Edelin as he carried out the operation. To all appearances, the fetus was dead. Doctor Edelin found no heartbeat and saw no other indication that he had a live being in his hands. If we give the prosecution the benefit of a remark by a defense witness that a test for heartbeat, to be absolutely conclusive, should extend longer than the few seconds testified to by Doctor Edelin, we have to note — besides the fact that there was no evidence as to any standard practice in this regard — that the witness did not say, nor could he say plausibly, that the test for the short period would be wanton or reckless behavior in any and all circumstances of a delivery. Here Doctor Gimenez, an eyewitness, joins in Doctor Edelin's observation. Doctor Gimenez testified: 'The baby [sic] was dead'; it 'had no signs of life, such as breathing or movement.' Doctor Gimenez had no criticism of the defendant on the score of his postnatal conduct.

* * *

"Manslaughter assumes that the victim was a live and independent person. This is well understood and the judge so charged. Destruction of a fetus *in utero* is not a manslaughter. The further question was debated at common law whether manslaughter might rest on a defendant's injuring a fetus *in utero*, where the fetus was later born alive, and then died of the injury without further guilty intervention by the defendant. In this Commonwealth, Holmes, J., seems to intimate a preference for the view that the prenatal acts could not ground a manslaughter despite the later live birth and death....

"...After *Wade-Bolton*, even if not before, the manslaughter statute could take hold only after a live birth and only with respect to acts of the physician in the postnatal period.

* * *

"The record shows that Doctor Edelin, as Chief Resident in OBS/GYN at Boston City Hospital, was well aware of the *Wade-Bolton* decisions and accordingly believed (correctly) that abortion was not automatically excluded at the stage of viability — that was for the Legislature to decide. He was concerned about viability, however, because it affected medical judgments and because he had a personal scruple against aborting a viable fetus.

"Again considering the evidence in a light favorable to the Commonwealth, there is nothing to impeach the defendant's good faith judgment that the particular fetus was nonviable, and nothing to suggest that that belief was grievously unreasonable by medical standards. An independent judgment would be required of Doctor Edelin as surgeon in the case, and his independent estimate of twenty to twenty-two weeks of gestation was consistent with the double-checked estimate of the experienced chief of clinic. The bona fides of Doctor Edelin's estimate is perhaps reinforced by the fact that he used a relatively small uterine incision. We find nothing in the course of the operation which might have alerted him to the probability that he had been mistaken in his estimate. It is not shown that he was mistaken in fact. Prosecution and defense experts divided on whether the fetus was viable, but a trier's belief in one set of experts would not begin to show that Doctor Edelin's judgment the other way was reckless. All the testimony bear comparison with the indication in *Wade* about a twenty-eight to twenty-four weeks gestational age in relation to viability. It is to be borne in mind, also, that no witness was prepared to state that this fetus had more than the remotest possibility of meaningful survival.

"If we accept, as we think we must, that there was nothing to show Doctor Edelin believed the fetus to be viable, or was flagrantly mistaken in believing it to be nonviable, then even a three to five minute wait after detachment of the placenta would not count as recklessness because Doctor Edelin would think it indifferent to the possibility of meaningful survival.

* * *

"...Here, however, we are able to say with confidence that on no acceptable standard was there proof sufficient to go to a jury. The defense has offered a proposed instruction drawing upon the definition of 'live-born infant' as formulated and published by the Committee on Terminology of the American College of Obstetricians and Gynecologists: 'LIVEBORN INFANT. Liveborn infant is a fetus, irrespective of its gestational age, that after complete expulsion or extraction from the mother, shows evidence of life—that is, heartbeats or respirations. Heartbeats are to be distinguished from several transient cardiac contractions; respirations are to be distinguished from fleeting respiratory efforts or gasps....' This suggested standard, which required a minimal demonstration of independent existence beyond 'fleeting respiratory efforts or gasps,' was less exacting proof and therefore more favorable from the Commonwealth's viewpoint than the standard that has been applied in practice around the country in manslaughter cases involving newborns. By this standard (as by any variant that might be considered acceptable) the Commonwealth failed in its proof.

* * *

"In the comparative calm of appellate review, the essential proposition emerges that the defendant on this record had no evil frame of mind, was actuated by no wanton or reckless acts in carrying out the medical procedures on October 3, 1973. A larger teaching of this case may be that, whereas a physician is accountable to the criminal law even when performing professional tasks, any assessment of his responsibility should pay due regard to the unavoidable difficulties and dubieties of many professional judgments.

"The judgment is reversed and the verdict set aside. Judgment of acquittal is to be entered.

"So ordered."

* * *

(The partial dissent of Justice Reardon and the partial dissent of Chief Justice Hennessey are deleted.)

QUESTIONS

1. May advances in medical technology endanger *Roe* in that viability may be moved so far back that only very early stage abortions will be allowed?
2. In effect, is the Court defining life?
3. If protected human life begins at conception, will hydraform moles (a relatively rare tumor that is a product of conception) be protected?
4. If *Roe* is overturned, is a stepping stone created for the loss of other constitutional rights?
5. With the Court's definition of manslaughter in *Edelin*, would it be possible for a physician to kill a viable fetus *in utero* and escape criminal liability?
6. Is the right to privacy a right invented by creative justices?
7. Should the Court recognize a fundamental right for abortions in the following cases:
   a) a fetus is found to have Down's syndrome;
   b) a couple cannot afford a baby;
   c) abortion is a convenient form of birth control;
   d) the fetus is female?

CHAPTER 2

GENETICS AND BIRTH CONTROL

INTRODUCTION

EFFORTS to restrict or regulate human reproduction have a long legal history in the United States. Early cases, *Buck v. Bell* (1927)[1] and *Skinner v. Oklahoma* (1942)[2] reflect the worst of the eugenics movement. Both of these cases dealt with sterilization statutes — one of a retarded girl and the other of a thief. Both statutes were based on biological misinformation. In *Buck*, it was assumed that Carrie Buck should be sterilized to prevent her from giving birth to a mentally retarded child. Oliver Wendell Holmes wrote, "three generations of imbeciles are enough."[3] The tragedy was that Carrie may not have been severely retarded, nor was her child.[4] Of course, even if it was likely that she would give birth to mentally retarded children, one may legitimately ask if the state should involuntarily sterilize her. *Skinner v. Oklahoma* reflects the same genetic control reasoning taken to absurd lengths. Oklahoma had a law which provided that certain types of habitual criminals could be sterilized. Underlying the law was a eugenic theory that assumed criminal traits were genetically transferred from parents to children. Thus, crime might be controlled by making it impossible for the criminal to produce offspring. Skinner was convicted of stealing chickens and of robbery, and, since it was his third offense, he was declared an habitual criminal and was subject to compulsory sterilization. Seemingly, Oklahoma feared that Skinner would produce children who, sharing his trait, would endanger chickens throughout the state. Unlike *Buck v. Bell*, the Supreme Court struck down the Oklahoma statute. Though reproductive privacy was mentioned in the opinion, the case centered on the idea that equal protection

---

[1] 274 U.S. 200 (1927).
[2] 316 U.S. 535 (1942).
[3] 274 U.S. at 207 (1927).
[4] Vose noted that after leaving the institution Carrie "married and settled down." Her child died at the age of nine and was reported to be "very bright." See, Vose, Clement E.: *Constitutional Change: Amendment Politics and Supreme Court Litigation Since 1900* (Lexington, Mass., Lexington, 1972, p. 15).

was denied. That is, while chicken thieves were subjected to sterilization, bank embezzlers were not. Such an arbitrary classification of criminal types, argued the Court, was irrational.

In the mid 1960s, the Court became concerned with laws that restricted the use of birth control; such laws were struck down as clear violations of reproductive privacy. More recently, artificial insemination has raised some significant legal questions. Artificial insemination is usually used to allow women to have children. These women, who for some reason, such as a husband who is sterile, would otherwise be unable to have children. It is estimated that between 6,000 and 10,000 artificial insemination by donor (AID) children are born annually in the United States. Donor insemination can be accomplished by using either fresh or frozen semen. Insemination occurs one to three times during ovulation. On the average, pregnancy occurs after insemination for 3.7 menstrual cycles.[5] The AID situations raise significant legal questions for all concerned. Yet, the legal status of AID is often poorly defined.

While AID is usually performed on women with sterile husbands, an increasing number of single women are seeking AID. Whether or not the woman is married, the law has recognized the woman who bears an AID child as the legal mother of the child. However, surrogate mothers have recently been used to bear an AID child. A surrogate mother might, for example, be used to bear a child for a couple who wishes children, but where the wife is unable to withstand pregnancy. In such a case, the surrogate mother might be artificially inseminated with semen provided by the husband of the woman unable to bear children. After the birth of the AID child, the surrogate would turn the child over to the couple.[6] Suppose, however, that the surrogate mother decides to keep the child? May she do so even if it negates a written contract?[7]

When the mother of an AID child is married and is inseminated with the husband's consent, there are unlikely to be serious legal problems. However, if that marriage later dissolves, questions might

[5]Curie-Cohen, Martin; Luttrell, Lisbeigh; and Shapiro, Sandra: Current practice of artificial insemination by donor in the United States (*New England Journal of Medicine,* 300:588, 1979).

[6]See generally, Keane, Noel P.: Legal problems of surrogate motherhood (*Southern Illinois University Law Journal,* 1980:147-169, 1980).

[7]"Whose Baby Is It, Anyway?" (*Newsweek,* 98:83, 1981). This case was terminated without a court judgment. Keane, Noel P. to senior author, personal communication, June 15, 1982.

be raised about paternity. Is the woman's husband the father of the child, even though the woman was impregnated with another man's sperm? Is the donor the legal father of the child? Would the AID child have a right to inherit from the donor or a right to be supported by the donor? Could the husband accuse the mother and AID donor of adultery? Currently, only fourteen states have statutes that address the status of husbands of women who have AID children.[8] Without statutes to govern, decisions are left to judicial discretion and judge-made law.

The child rarely learns that he/she is an AID child. Many physicians even try to match the physical appearance of the semen donor and the husband. Finegold notes a family with four AID children, all with different donors, yet with no suspicion of AID origins by friends, relatives, or pediatricians.[9] In many states, questions of legitimacy and inheritance rights of AID children remain to be resolved. While screening for a match in physical appearance between donor and husband is common, many physicians do little if any genetic screening. There have been instances of AID children being born with preventable genetic defects.[10] There is an increasing problem with multiple paternity by donors. Few physicians have policies concerning maximum use of a donor. Yet, as the number of AID births continues to increase, the frequent use of the same donors increases the likelihood of consanguinity. Especially in smaller communities where a physician frequently uses the same donor, there is a chance that AID children will marry who have the same donor parent. These consanguinity problems are complicated by the practice of physician's maintaining limited records pertaining to AID, and it is doubtful that physicians will keep records on the outcomes of AID pregnancies.[11] Physician failure to perform genetic screening and failure to use multiple donors opens up significant possibilities for legal action against physicians.

[8]Curie-Cohen, op cit., p. 587.

[9]Finegold, Wilfred J.:*Artificial Insemination,* 2nd ed. (Springfield, Thomas, 1976, p. 33).

[10]Curie-Cohen, op cit., pp. 585-590.

[11]Shapiro, David N., and Hutchison, Raymond J.: Familial histiocytosis in offspring of two pregnancies after artificial insemination (*New England Journal of Medicine, 304*:757-759, 1981); Johnson, William G.; Schwartz, Robin C.; and Chutorian, Abe M.:Artificial insemination by donors: The need for genetic screening (*New England Journal of Medicine, 304*:755-757, 1981).

Recently, genetic experimentation has raised concerns about the dangers that experimental errors might pose to existing life forms. Although such questions may seem more in the realm of fiction than reality, new life forms have already been created and patented.[12] As we move into the twenty-first century, cloning of higher life forms, genetic manipulation aimed at creating "super humans," and creation of a subhuman species become increasingly real possibilities.[13]

---

[12]*Diamond v. Chakrabarty*, 447 U.S. 303 (1980).
[13]See generally, Ramsey, Paul:*Fabricated Man* (New Haven, Yale, 1970).

BUCK V. BELL

(U.S. Supreme Court, 1927)
274 U.S. 200

Carrie Buck, a "feeble minded" female, daughter of a feeble minded female, and herself mother of an illegitimate feeble minded child was sterilized by court order. Is forced sterilization of mental defectives constitutional?

MR. JUSTICE OLIVER HOLMES FOR THE COURT:

* * *

"...There can be no doubt that so far as procedure is concerned the rights of the patient are most carefully considered, and as every step in this case was taken in scrupulous compliance with the statute and after months of observation, there is no doubt that in that respect the plaintiff in error has had due process at law.

"The attack is not upon the procedure but upon the substantive law. It seems to be contended that in no circumstances could such an order be justified. It certainly is contended that the order cannot be justified upon the existing grounds. The judgment finds the facts that have been recited and that Carrie Buck is the probable potential parent of socially inadequate offspring, like-wise afflicted, that she may be sexually sterilized without detriment to her general health and that her welfare and that of society will be promoted by her sterilization, and thereupon makes the order. In view of the general declarations of the Legislature and the specific findings of the Court obviously we cannot say as matter of law that the grounds do not exist, and if they exist they justify the result. We have seen more than once that the public welfare may call upon the best citizens for their lives. It would be strange if it could not call upon those who already sap the strength of the State for these lesser sacrifices, often not felt to be such by those concerned, in order to prevent our being swamped with incompetence. It is better for all the world, if instead of waiting to execute degenerate offspring for crime, or to let them starve for their imbecility, society can prevent those who are manifestly unfit from continuing their kind. The principle that sustains compulsory vaccination is broad enough to cover cutting the Fallopian tubes.... Three generations of imbeciles are enough."

* * *

(Justice Pierce Butler dissented.)

SKINNER V. OKLAHOMA

(U.S. Supreme Court, 1942)
316 U.S. 535

May an habitual criminal be sterilized?

MR. JUSTICE DOUGLAS FOR THE COURT:

* * *

"The statute involved is Oklahoma's Habitual Criminal Sterilization Act.... That Act defines an 'habitual criminal' as a person who,
having been convicted two or more times for crimes 'amounting to
felonies involving moral turpitude' either in an Oklahoma court or
in a court of any other State, is thereafter convicted of such a felony
in Oklahoma and is sentenced to a term of imprisonment in an
Oklahoma penal institution.... Machinery is provided for the institution by the Attorney General of a proceeding against such a person in the Oklahoma courts for a judgment that such person shall be
rendered sexually sterile....

"...Only one other provision of the Act is material here and that is
section 195 which provides that 'offenses arising out of the violation
of the prohibitory laws, revenue acts, embezzlement, or political offenses, shall not come or be considered within the terms of this Act.'

Petitioner was convicted in 1926 of the crime of stealing chickens
and was sentenced to the Oklahoma State Reformatory. In 1929 he
was convicted of the crime of robbery with firearms and was sentenced to the reformatory. In 1934 he was convicted again of robbery
with firearms and was sentenced to the penitentiary. He was confined there in 1935 when the Act was passed. In 1936 the Attorney
General instituted proceedings against him. Petitioner in his answer
challenged the Act as unconstitutional by reason of the Fourteenth
Amendment. A jury trial was had. The court instructed the jury that
the crimes of which petitioner had been convicted were felonies involving moral turpitude and that the only question for the jury was
whether the operation of vasectomy could be performed on petitioner without detriment to his general health. The jury found that it
could be. A judgment directing that the operation of vasectomy be
performed on petitioner was affirmed by the Supreme Court of
Oklahoma by a five to four decision...."

"Several objections to the constitutionality of the Act have been pressed upon us. It is urged that the Act cannot be sustained as an exercise of the police power in view of the state of scientific authorities respecting inheritability of criminal traits. It is argued that due process is lacking because under this Act, unlike the act upheld in *Buck v. Bell...*, the defendant is given no opportunity to be heard on the issue as to whether he is the probably potential parent of socially undesirable character and that the sterilization provided for is cruel and unusual punishment and violative of the Fourteenth Amendment.... We pass those points without intimating an opinion on them, for there is a feature of the act which clearly condemns it. That is its failure to meet the requirements of the equal protection clause of the Fourteenth Amendment.

"We do not stop to point out all of the inequalities in this Act. A few examples will suffice. In Oklahoma grand larceny is a felony.... Larceny is grand larceny when the property taken exceeds $20 in value.... Embezzlement is punishable "in the manner prescribed for feloniously stealing property of the value of that embezzled...." Hence he who embezzles property worth more than $20 is guilty of a felony. A clerk who appropriates over $20 from his employer's till ...and a stranger who steals the same amount are thus both guilty of felonies. If the latter repeats his act and is convicted three times, he may be sterilized. But the clerk is not subject to the pains and penalities of the Act no matter how large his embezzlements nor how frequent his convictions. A person who enters a chicken coop and steals chickens commits a felony...and he may be sterilized if he is thrice convicted. If, however, he is a bailee of the property and fraudulently appropriates it, he is an embezzler.... Hence no matter how habitual his proclivities for embezzlement are and no matter how often his conviction, he may not be sterilized....

***

"...We are dealing here with legislation which involves one of the basic civil rights of man. Marriage and procreation are fundamental to the very existence and survival of the race. The power to sterilize, if exercised, may have subtle, far-reaching and devastating effects. In evil or reckless hands it can cause races or types which are inimical to the dominant group to wither and disappear. There is no redemption for the individual whom the law touches. Any experiment which the State conducts is to his irreparable injury. He is forever deprived of a basic liberty.... We advert to them merely in emphasis of our view that strict scrutiny of the classification which a State makes in a sterilization law is essential, lest unwittingly or otherwise invidious discriminations are made against groups or types of individuals in violation of the constitutional guaranty of just and equal laws.... When the law lays an unequal hand on those who have committed intrinsically the same quality of offense and sterilizes one and not the other, it has made as an invidious a discrimination as if it had selected a particular race of nationality for oppressive treatment.... Sterilization of those who . . thrice committed grand larceny . . is a clear, pointed, unmistakable discrimination...."

***

CHIEF JUSTICE STONE CONCURRING:

***

"...I think the real question we have to consider is not one of equal protection, but whether the wholesale condemnation of a class to such an invasion of personal liberty without opportunity to any individual to show that his is not the type of case which would justify resort to it, satisfies the demands of due process.

"...Although petitioner here was given a hearing to ascertain whether sterilization would be detrimental to his health, he was given none to discover whether his criminal tendencies are of an inheritable type. Undoubtedly a state may, after appropriate inquiry, constitutionally, interfere with the personal liberty of the individual to prevent the transmission by inheritance of his socially injurious tendencies....

"...But the State does not contend—nor can there be any pretense—that either common knowledge or experience, or scientific investigation, has given assurance that the criminal tendencies of any class of habitual offenders are universally or even generally inheritable. In such circumstances, inquiry whether such is the fact in the case of any particular individual cannot rightly be dispensed with..."

JUSTICE JACKSON CONCURRING:

***

"I also think the present plan to sterilize the individual in pursuit of a eugenic plan to eliminate from the race characteristics that are only vaguely identified and which in our present state of knowledge are uncertain as to transmissibility presents other constitutional questions of gravity. This Court has sustained such an experiment with respect to an imbecile, a person with definite and observable characteristics where the condition had persisted through three generations and afforded grounds for the belief that it was transmissible and would continue to manifest itself in generations to come....

There are limits to the extent to which a legislatively represented majority may conduct biological experiments at the expense of the dignity and personality and natural powers of a minority — even those who have been guilty of what the majority define as crimes. But this Act falls down before reaching this problem, which I mention only to avoid the implication that such a question may not exist because not discussed. On it I would also reserve judgment."

IN RE CAVITT

(Supreme Court of Nebraska, 1968)
157 N. W. 2d 171

Thirty-five-year-old Gloria Cavitt, mother of eight, having been confined to a home for the mentally deficient, could not be released without undergoing sterilization. May the state sterilize the mentally deficient?

MR. JUSTICE CARTER FOR THE COURT:

"The primary question before this court is the constitutionality of [a law]...which states: 'It shall be the duty of the board of examiners to make a psychiatric and physical examination of these patients and, if after a careful examination, such board of examiners finds that such patient is mentally deficient, in the opinion of the board of examiners, is apparently capable of bearing or begetting offspring and, based on their psychiatric and medical findings as a result of this examination, it is the opinion of the board of examiners that such patient should be sterilized, as a condition prerequisite to the parole or discharge, then such patient shall not be paroled or discharged, as the case may be, unless said patient be made sterile, and that such operation be performed for the prevention of procreation as in the judgment of the board of examiners would be most appropriate to each individual case.'

"It will be noted that the findings of the board of examiners necessary to make an order for the sexual sterilization of a mentally defective patient are: (1) That the patient is mentally deficient, (2) that the patient is apparently capable of bearing or begetting offspring, and (3) that in its opinion such patient should be sterilized as a condition to parole or discharge. It is the contention of Gloria that the power to sexually sterilize a mentally deficient patient exists only when it is determined that the mental deficiency is such that it will be inherited by offspring. The statute does not require any such finding by the board nor does the evidence support any such finding. Under such circumstances it is asserted that the applicable statute does not contain adequate standards for the guidance of the board of examiners and by its terms permits arbitrary action by such board in such degree as to render the act unconstitutional as an unlawful delegation of legislative power.

***

"The testimony of the two psychiatrists, the psychologist, and the general medical practitioner, all members of the board, can be summarized as follows: Gloria has an IQ of 71 and is in the lower 2 or 3 percent of the population in intelligence. All agreed that she was mentally deficient and probably capable of bearing children. After a review of Gloria's record and the observation of her, plus the IQ test, it was determined that she lacked the mental stability to handle social adjustment problems. Her attitude and personal feelings were considered. Consideration was given to the probable effect upon her of having more children, her minimal capacity to handle the responsibilities of parenthood, the possibility of producing mentally defective children, and the probability that added responsibilities of parenthood would in all likelihood handicap her potential rehabilitation.

***

"Sterilization is a much misunderstood subject when applied to the mentally deficient. The public has a natural revulsion of feeling against sterilization of mental defectives even when it is clear that the public welfare requires it. Mental deficiency with its alarming results presents a social and economic problem of grave importance which gives rise to the exercise of the police power by the Legislature.... Thus far we have been endeavoring to demonstrate that the statute under consideration, measured by the purpose for which it was enacted and the conditions which warranted it, and justified by the findings of experts in biological science, is a proper and reasonable exercise of the police power. The opposition to such a statute as we have before us is largely based on the assumption that the operation is inhuman, unreasonable, and oppressive. The surgical operation of vasectomy on mentally defective males and of salpingectomy on mentally defective females is a simple operation without pain or discomfort to the patient. It does not reduce his sex impulses nor limit his capacity to engage in sexual relations. It does no harm to the patient other than to eliminate his capacity to procreate.

"We limit our holding to the facts of this case and the statute we have before us. We have here a case where the patient has not been cured, but who is eligible for release from the home if she is sterilized. Sterilization is only a condition for parole or discharge. It is compulsory only if she insists upon her release. We fail to see how the statute is in any manner unconstitutional on any grounds under these precise circumstances. It constitutes a reasonable invocation of the police power for the public welfare...."

***

(Justices Smith, McCown, Newton, and Boslaugh dissented.)

GRISWOLD V. STATE OF CONNECTICUT

(U.S. Supreme Court, 1965)
381 U.S. 479

May a state forbid the use of birth control by married persons?

Mr. Justice Douglas Delivered the Opinion of the Court:

"Appellant Griswold is Executive Director of the Planned Parenthood League of Connecticut. Appellant Buston is a licensed physician and a professor at the Yale Medical School who served as Medical Director for the League at its Center in New Haven—a center open and operating from November 1 to November 10, 1961, when appellants were arrested.

"They gave information, instruction, and medical advice to *married persons* [Court's emphasis] as to the means of preventing conception. They examined the wife and prescribed the best contraceptive device or materials for her use. Fees were usually charged, although some couples were serviced free.

"The statutes whose constitutionality is involved in this appeal...[provides]: 'Any persons who uses any drug, medicinal article or instrument for the purpose of preventing conception shall be fined not less than fifty dollars or imprisoned not less than sixty days nor more than one year or be both fined and imprisoned.... Any person who assists, abets, counsels, causes, hires or commands another to commit any offense may be prosecuted and punished as if he were the principal offender.'

"The appellants were found guilty as accessories and fined $100 each....

***

"...We do not sit as a super-legislature to determine the wisdom, need, and propriety of laws that touch economic problems, business affairs, or social conditions. This law, however, operates directly on an intimate relation of husband and wife and their physician's role in one aspect of that relation.

"The association of people is not mentioned in the Constitution nor the Bill of Rights. The right to educate a child in a school of the parents' choice — whether public or private or parochial — is also not mentioned. Nor is the right to study any particular subject or any foreign language. Yet the First Amendment has been construed to include certain of those rights.

***

"...[W]e protected the 'freedom to associate and privacy in one's associations,' noting that freedom of association was a peripheral First Amendment right. Disclosure of membership lists of a constitutionally valid association, we held, was invalid 'as entailing the likelihood of a substantial restraint upon the exercise by petitioner's members of their right to freedom of association....' In other words, the First Amendment has a penumbra where privacy is protected from government intrusion. In like context, we have protected forms of 'association' that are not political in the customary sense but pertain to the social, legal, and economic benefit of the members....

***

"The foregoing cases suggest that specific guarantees in the Bill of Rights have penumbras, formed by emanations from those guarantees that help give them life and substance.... Various guarantees create zones of privacy. The right of association contained in the penumbra of the First Amendment is one, as we have seen. The Third Amendment in its prohibition against the quartering of soldiers 'in any house' in time of peace without the consent of the owner is another facet of that privacy. The Fourth Amendment explicitly affirms the 'right of the people to be secure in their persons, houses, papers, and effects, against unreasonable searches and seizures.' The Fifth Amendment in its Self-Incrimination Clause enables the citizen to create a zone of privacy which government may not force him to surrender to his detriment. The Ninth Amendment provides: 'The enumeration in the Constitution, of certain rights, shall not be construed to deny or disparage others retained by the people.'

***

"The present case, then, concerns a relationship lying within the zone of privacy created by several fundamental constitutional guarantees. And it concerns a law which, in forbidding the use of contraceptives rather than regulating their manufacture or sale, seeks to achieve its goals by means having a maximum destructive impact upon that relationship. Such a law cannot stand in light of the familiar principle, so often applied by this Court, that a 'governmental purpose to control or prevent activities constitutionally subject to state regulation may not be achieved by means which sweep unnecessarily broadly and thereby invade the area of protected freedoms....' Would we allow the police to search the sacred precincts of marital bedrooms for telltale signs of the use of contraceptives? The very idea is repulsive to the notions of privacy surrounding the marriage relationship.

"We deal with a right of privacy older than the Bill of Rights — older than our political parties, older than our school system. Marriage is a coming together for better or for worse, hopefully enduring, and intimate to the degree of being sacred. It is an association that promotes a way of life, not causes; a harmony in living, not political faiths; a bilateral loyalty, not commercial or social projects. Yet it is an association for as noble a purpose as any involved in our prior decisions.

"Reversed."

MR. JUSTICE GOLDBERG, WHOM THE CHIEF JUSTICE AND MR. JUSTICE BRENNAN JOIN, CONCURRING:

***

"I agree with the Court that Connecticut's birth-control law un-constitutionally intrudes upon the right of marital privacy, and I join in its opinion and judgment.... [T]he concept of liberty protects those personal rights that are fundamental, and is not confined to the specific terms of the Bill of Rights. My conclusion that the con-cept of liberty is not so restricted and that it embraces the right of marital privacy though that right is not mentioned explicitly in the Constitution is supported both by numerous decisions of this Court, referred to in the Court's opinion, and by the language and history of the Ninth Amendment....

***

"...The language and history of the Ninth Amendment reveal that the Framers of the Constitution believed that there are addi-tional fundamental rights, protected from governmental infringe-ment, which exist alongside those fundamental rights specifically mentioned in the first eight constitutional amendments.

"The Ninth Amendment reads, 'The enumeration in the Consti-tution, of certain rights, shall not be construed to deny or disparage others retained by the people.' The Amendment is almost entirely the work of James Madison. It was introduced in Congress by him and passed the House and Senate with little or no debate and vir-tually no change in language. It was proffered to quiet expressed fears that a bill of specifically enumerated rights could not be suffi-ciently broad to cover all essential rights and that the specific men-tion of certain rights would be interpreted as a denial that others were protected.

***

"While this Court has had little occasion to interpret the Ninth Amendment, 'It cannot be presumed that any clause in the Constitu-tion is intended to be without effect....' The Ninth Amendment to the Constitution may be regarded by some as a recent discovery and may be forgotten by others, but since 1791 it has been a basic part of the Constitution which we are sworn to uphold. To hold that a right so basic and fundamental and so deep-rooted in our society as the right of privacy in marriage may be infringed because that right is not guaranteed in so many words by the first eight amendments to the Constitution is to ignore the Ninth Amendment and to give it no effect whatsoever...."

***

MR. JUSTICE HARLAN, CONCURRING IN THE JUDGMENT:

***

"In my view, the proper constitutional inquiry in this case is whether this Connecticut statute infringes the Due Process Clause of the Fourteenth Amendment because the enactment violates basic values 'implicit in the concept of ordered liberty....' While the relevant inquiry may be aided by resort to one or more of the provisions of the Bill of Rights, it is not dependent on them or any of their radiations. The Due Process Clause of the Fourteenth Amendment stands, in my opinion, on its own bottom."

***

(The concurrence of Justice White is omitted.)

MR. JUSTICE BLACK, WITH WHOM MR. JUSTICE STEWART JOINS, DISSENTING:

***

"...In order that there may be no room at all to doubt why I vote as I do, I feel constrained to add that the law is every bit as offensive to me as it is my Brethren of the majority and my Brothers Harlan, White and Goldberg who, reciting reasons why it is offensive to them, hold it unconstitutional....

"...The two defendants here were active participants in an organization which gave physical examinations to women, advised them what kind of contraceptive devices or medicines would most likely be satisfactory for them, and then supplied the devices themselves, all for a graduated scale of fees, based on the family income. Thus these defendants admittedly engaged with others in a planned course of conduct to help people violate the Connecticut law. Merely because some speech was used in carrying on the conduct — just as in ordinary life some speech accompanies most kinds of conduct — we are not in my view justified in holding that the First Amendment forbids the State to punish their conduct. Strongly as I desire to protect all First Amendment freedoms, I am unable to stretch the Amendment so as to afford protection to the conduct of these defendants in violating the Connecticut law...."

* * *

"One of the most effective ways of diluting or expanding a constitutionally guaranteed right is to substitute for the crucial word or words of a constitutional guarantee another word or words, more or less flexible and more or less restricted in meaning. This fact is well illustrated by the use of the term 'right of privacy' as a comprehensive substitute for the Fourth Amendment's guarantee against 'unreasonable searches and seizures.' 'Privacy' is a broad, abstract and ambiguous concept which can easily be shrunken in meaning but which can also, on the other hand, easily be interpreted as a constitutional ban against many things other than searches and seizures. I have expressed the view many times that First Amendment freedoms, for example, have suffered from a failure of the courts to stick to the simple language of the First Amendment in construing it, instead of invoking multitudes of words substituted for those the Framers used.... for these reasons I get nowhere in this case by talk about a constitutional 'right of privacy' as an emanation from one or more constitutional provisions. I like my privacy as well as the next one, but I am nevertheless compelled to admit that government has a right to invade it unless prohibited by some specific constitutional provision...."

* * *

"The due process argument which my Brothers Harlan and White adopt here is based...on the premise that this Court is vested with power to invalidate all state laws that it considers to be arbitrary, capricious, unreasonable, or oppressive, or this Court's belief that a particular state law under scrutiny has no 'rational or justifying' purpose, or is offensive to a 'sense of fairness and justice....' While I completely subscribe to the holding of *Marbury v. Madison*...and subsequent cases, that our Court has constitutional power to strike down statutes, state or federal, that violate commands of the Federal Constitution, I do not believe that we are granted power by the Due Process Clause or any other constitutional provision or provisions to measure constitutionally by our belief that legislation...is offensive to our own notions of 'civilized standards of conduct.' Such an appraisal of the wisdom of legislation is an attribute of the power to make laws, not of the power to interpret them. The use by federal courts of such a formula or doctrine or whatnot to veto federal or state laws simply takes away from Congress and States the power to make laws based on their own judgment of fairness and wisdom and transfers that power to this Court for ultimate determination—a power which was specifically denied to federal courts by the convention that framed the Constitution.

* * *

"My Brother Goldberg has adopted the recent discovery that the Ninth Amendment as well as the Due Process Clause can be used by this Court as authority to strike down all state legislation which this Court thinks violates 'fundamental principles of liberty and justice,' or is contrary to the 'traditions and (collective) consciences of our people....' [O]ne would certainly have to look far beyond the language of the Ninth Amendment to find that the Framers vested in this Court any such awesome veto powers over lawmaking, either by the States or by the Congress. Nor does anything in the history of the Amendment offer any support for such a shocking doctrine. The whole history of the adoption of the Constitution and Bill of Rights points the other way.... That Amendment was passed, not to broaden the powers of this Court or any other department of the General Government, but, as every student of history knows, to assure the people that the Constitution in all its provisions was intended to limit the Federal Government to the powers granted expressly or by necessary implication. If any broad, unlimited power to hold laws unconstitutional because they offend what this Court conceives to be the '(collective) conscience of our people' is vested in this Court by the Ninth Amendment, the Fourteenth Amendment, or any other provision of the Constitution, it was not given by the Framers, but rather has been bestowed on the Court by the Court. This fact is perhaps responsible for the peculiar phenomenon that for a period of a century and a half no serious suggestion was ever made that the Ninth Amendment, enacted to protect state powers against federal invasion, could be used as a weapon of federal power to prevent state legislatures from passing laws they consider appropriate to govern local affairs. Use of any such broad, unbounded judicial authority would make of this Court's members a day-to-day constitutional convention.

* * *

"...So far as I am concerned, Connecticut's law as applied here is not forbidden by any provision of the Federal Constitution as that

Constitution was written, and I would therefore affirm."

(A dissenting opinion by Justice Stewart, which Justice Black joined, is omitted.)

PEOPLE V. SORENSEN

(Supreme Court of California, 1968)
437 P. 2d 495

Is the husband of a woman who conceived a child through AID legally responsible for support of the child?

McComb, Justice:

"Defendant appeals from a judgment convicting him of violating section 270 of the Penal Code (willful failure to provide for his minor child), a misdemeanor.

"The settled statement of facts recites that seven years after defendant's marriage it was medically determined that he was sterile. His wife desired a child, either by artificial insemination or by adoption, and at first defendant refused to consent. About 15 years after the marriage defendant agreed to the artificial insemination of his wife. Husband and wife, then residents of San Joaquin County, consulted a physician in San Francisco. They signed an agreement, which is on the letterhead of the physician, requesting the physician to inseminate the wife with the sperm of a white male. The semen was to be selected by the physician, and under no circumstances were the parties to demand the name of the donor.... The physician treated Mrs. Sorensen, and she became pregnant....

"A male child was born to defendant's wife in San Joaquin County on October 14, 1960. The information for the birth certificate was given by the mother, who named defendant as the father. Defendant testified that he had not provided the information on the birth certificate and did not recall seeing it before the trial.

"For about four years the family had a normal family relationship, defendant having represented to friends that he was the child's father and treated the boy as his son. In 1964, Mrs. Sorensen separated from defendant and moved to Sonoma County with the boy. At separation, Mrs. Sorensen told defendant that she wanted no support for the boy, and she consented that a divorce be granted to defendant. Defendant obtained a decree of divorce, which recites that the court retained 'jurisdiction regarding the possible obligation of plaintiff in regard to a minor child born to defendant.'

"In the summer of 1966 when Mrs. Sorensen became ill and could not work, she applied for public assistance under the Aid to Needy Children program. The County of Sonoma supplied this aid until Mrs. Sorensen was able to resume work. Defendant paid no support for the child since the separation in 1964, although demand therefore was made by the district attorney. The municipal court found defendant guilty of violating section 270 of the Penal Code and granted him probation for three years on condition that he make payments of $50 per month for support through the district attorney's office.

* * *

"Is the husband of a woman, who with his consent was artificially inseminated with semen of a third-party donor, guilty of the crime of failing to support a child who is the product of such insemination, in violation of section 270 of the Penal Code? [Court's emphasis.] The law is that the defendant is the lawful father of the child born to his wife, which child was conceived by artificial insemination to which he consented, and his conduct carries with it an obligation of support within the meaning of section 270 of the Penal Code.

"Under the facts of this case, the term 'father' as used in section 270 cannot be limited to the biologic or natural father as those terms are generally understood. The determinative factor is whether the legal relationship of father and child exists. A child conceived through heterologous artificial insemination does not have a 'natural father,' as that term is commonly used. The anonymous donor of the sperm cannot be considered the 'natural father,' as he is no more responsible for the use made of his sperm than is the donor of blood or a kidney.... With the use of frozen semen, the donor may even be dead at the time the semen is used. Since there is no 'natural father,' we can only look for a lawful father.

* * *

"...In determining whether a penal statute is sufficiently explicit to inform those who are subject to it what is required of them, the court must endeavor, if possible, to view the statute from the standpoint of a reasonable man who might be subject to its terms....

"In light of these principles of statutory construction, a reasonable man who because of his inability to procreate actively participates and consents to his wife's artificial insemination in the hope that a child will be produced whom they will treat as their own, knows that such behavior carries with it the legal responsibilities of fatherhood and criminal responsibility for nonsupport. One who consents to the production of a child cannot create a temporary relation to be assumed and disclaimed at will, but the arrangement must be of such character as to impose an obligation of supporting those for whose existence he is directly responsible. As noted by the trial court, it is safe to assume that without defendant's active participation and consent the child would not have been procreated.

***

"The question of the liability of the husband for support of a child created through artificial insemination is one of first impression in this state and has been raised in only a few cases outside the state, none of them involving a criminal prosecution for failure to provide. Although other courts considering the question have found some existing legal theory to hold the 'father' responsible, results have varied on the question of legitimacy. In *Gursky v. Gursky*...the court held that the child was illegitimate but that the husband was liable for the child's support because consent to the insemination implied a promise to support.

"In *Strnad v. Strnad*...the court found that a child conceived through artificial insemination was not illegitimate and granted visitation rights to the husband in a custody proceeding.

It is less crucial to determine the status of the child than the status of defendant as the father. Categorizing the child as either legitimate or illegitimate does not resolve the issue of the legal consequences flowing from defendant's participation in the child's existence. Under our statute, both legitimate and illegitimate minors have a right to support from their parents....

***

"The public policy of this state favors legitimation...and no valid public purpose is served by stigmatizing an artificially conceived child as illegitimate An illegitimate child is 'one not recognized by law as lawful offspring; born of parents not married to each other; conceived in fornication or adultery...; illegitimacy is defined as 'the state or condition of one whose parents were not married at the time of his birth....'

"In the absence of legislation prohibiting artificial insemination, the offspring of defendant's valid marriage to the child's mother was lawfully begotten and was not the product of an illicit or adulterous relationship. Adultry is defined as 'the voluntary sexual intercourse of a married person with a person other than the offender's husband or wife....' Since the doctor may be a woman, or the husband himself may administer the insemination by a syringe, this is patently absurd; to consider it an act of adultery with the donor, who at the time of insemination may be a thousand miles away or may even be dead, is equally absurd. Nor are we persuaded that the concept of legitimacy demands that the child be the actual offspring of the husband of the mother and if semen of some other male is utilized the resulting child is illegitimate.

"In California, legitimacy is a legal status that may exist despite the fact that the husband is not the natural father of the child.... The Legislature has provided for legitimation of a child born before wedlock by the subsequent marriage of its parents..., for legitimation by acknowledgment by the father..., and for inheritance rights of illegitimates..., and since the subject of legitimation as well as that of succession of property is properly one for legislative action..., we are not required in this case to do more than decide that, within the meaning of the section 270 of the Penal Code, defendant is the lawful father of the child conceived through heterologous artificial insemination and born during his marriage to the child's mother.

"The judgment is affirmed.

Traynor, C.J., and Peters, Tobriner, Mosk, Burke, and Sullivan, J.J., concur."

IN RE ADOPTION OF ANONYMOUS

(Surrogate's Court, Kings County, 1973)
74 Misc. 2d 99

Is the former husband of a woman who bore an AID child a parent of the child and must his consent be obtained for the adoption of the child by another?

SURROGATE JUDGE NATHAN R. SOBEL:

"...During the marriage the child was born of consensual AID. The husband was listed as the father on the birth certificate. Later the couple separated and the separation was followed by a divorce. Both the separation agreement and the divorce decree declare the child to be the 'daughter' and 'child' of the couple. The wife was granted support and the husband visitation rights. He has faithfully visited and performed all the support conditions of the decree. The wife later remarried and her new husband is petitioning to adopt the child. The first husband has refused his consent. Confronted with that legal impediment, the peititioner has suggested that the first husband's consent is not required since he is not the 'parent' of the child.

* * *

"New York has a strong policy in favor of legitimacy. This is evidenced by the recent enactment of section 24 of the Domestic Relations Law.... Under that statute a child born of a void...or voidable...marriage, even if the marriage is deliberately and knowingly bigamous, incestuous or adulterous, is legitimate and entitled to all the rights (inheritance, support, etc.) of a child born during a perfectly valid marriage. In the face of the liberal policy expressed by such a statute, it would seem absurd to hold illegitimate a child born during a valid marriage, of parents desiring but unable to conceive a child and both consenting and agreeing to the impregnation of the mother by a carefully and medically selected anonymous donor.

"It must be recognized that there exist moral and religious objections to artificial insemination.... But these are stronger against bigamous, incestuous and adulterous relationships. That such objections have not prevented as a matter of state policy the legitimation of the children of such marriages, establishes that our liberal policy is for the protection of the child, not the parents. It serves no purpose whatsoever to stigmatize the AID child; or to compel the parents formally to adopt in order to confer upon the AID child the status and rights of a naturally conceived child.

"It is determined that a child born of consensual AID during a valid marriage is a legitimate child entitled to the rights and privileges of a naturally conceived child of the same marriage. The father of such child is therefore the 'parent'...whose consent is required to the adoption of such child by another.

"The petition for adoption of the child by the stepfather must be dismissed."

C. M. V. C. C.

(Juvenile and Domestic Relations Court
Cumberland County, New Jersey, 1977).
377 A 2d. 821

May a semen donor obtain visitation rights with respect to a child born as a result of artificial insemination?

JUDGE TESTA:

***

"...C.C. testified that she has been discussing with C.M. the possibility of having a child by artificial insemination, inquiring of him whether she should ask one of his friends to supply the sperm. C.M. suggested that he provide it and C.C. agreed to his suggestion. C.M. testified that he and C.C. had been seeing each other for some time and were contemplating marriage. She wanted a child and wanted him to be the father, but did not want to have intercourse with him before their marriage. Therefore, he agreed to provide the sperm.

***

"Over a period of several months, C.C. went to C.M.'s apartment where they attempted the artificial insemination. C.M. would stay in one room while C.C. went to another room to attempt to inseminate herself with semen provided by C.M. After several attempts over a period of several months, C.C. did conceive a child.

"C.M. testified that until C.C. was about three months pregnant, he assumed he would act toward the child in the same manner as most fathers act toward their children. C.C. denies this, testifying that C.M. was to be only a visitor in her home — much as any of her other friends. In either case, at that point the relationship between C.M. and C.C. broke off. This present application is a request by C.M. for visitation rights to the baby. His request is strenuously opposed by C.C.

***

"...There is no married couple. There is no anonymous donor. Rather, we have a woman who chooses to have a baby and a man who chooses to provide the needed sperm, who are not married to each other and who choose a method of conception other than sexual intercourse. If the conception took place by intercourse, there would be no question that the 'donor' would be the father. The issue becomes whether a man is any less a father because he provides the semen by a method different from that normally used.

***

"The courts have consistently shown a policy favoring the requirement that a child be provided with a father as well as a mother. In a situation where there is an anonymous donor the courts have required that the person who consents to the use of sperm, not his own, be responsible for fathering the child.

"In this case there is a known man who is the donor. There is no husband. If the couple had been married and the husband's sperm was used artificially, he would be considered the father. If a woman conceives a child by intercourse, the 'donor' who is not married to the mother is no less a father than the man who is married to the mother. Likewise, if an unmarried woman conceives a child through artificial insemination from semen from a known man, that man cannot be considered to be less a father because he is not married to the woman.

"When a husband consents to his wife's artificial insemination from an anonymous donor, he takes upon himself the responsibilities of fatherhood. By donating his semen anonymously, the donor impliedly gives it without taking on such responsibilities for its use. But here C.C. received semen from C.M. who was a friend—someone she had known for at least two years. The court finds that the evidence supports C.M.'s contention that he and C.C. had a long-standing dating relationship and he fully intended to assume the responsibilities of parenthood. There was no one else who was in a position to take upon himself the responsibilities of fatherhood when the child was conceived. The evidence does not adequately support C.C.'s contention, as argued by her attorney in his brief and stated in her testimony, that C.M. waived his parental rights.

"It is in a child's best interests to have two parents whenever possible. The court takes no position as to the propriety of the use of artificial insemination between unmarried persons, but must be concerned with the best interest of the child in granting custody or visitation, and for such consideration will not make a distinction between a child conceived naturally or artificially.... In this situation a man wants to take upon himself the responsibility of being a father to a child he is responsible for helping to conceive. The evidence does not support C.C.'s argument that he is unfit. The evidence demonstrates that C.M. attempted to establish a relationship with the child but was thwarted in his attempts by C.C. Contrary to C.C.'s argument, C.M. has shown a genuine interest in the child; he is a teacher and educationally able to aid his development, and is financially capable of contributing to his support. C.M.'s consent and active participation in the procedure leading to conception should place upon him the responsibilities of fatherhood. The court will not deny him the privileges of fatherhood. His motion for the right of visitation is granted...."

* * *

DOE V. ATTORNEY GENERAL

(Michigan Court of Appeals, 1981)
106 Mich App 169

Is there a constitutional right to hire the services of a surrogate mother?

JUDGE M. J. KELLY:

"In this case, we are asked to declare unconstitutional those sections of the Michigan Adoption Code...which prohibit the exchange of money or other consideration in connection with adoption and related proceedings....

"Jane Doe and John Doe are pseudonyms for a married couple residing in Wayne County....

"It is alleged that Jane Doe has undergone a tubal ligation, rendering her bilogically incapable of bearing children and that the Does 'wish to have a child biologically related to John Doe.' Mary Roe is employed as a secretary by John Doe and also resides in

Wayne County. The complaint alleges that these parties contemplate and intend to enter into the following agreement:

(a)That Jane Doe and John Doe will pay Mary Roe a sum of money in consideration for her promise to bear and deliver John Doe's child by means of artificial insemination.

(b)That a licensed physician will conduct the artificial insemination process.

(c)That prior to the delivery of said child, John Doe will file a notice of intent to claim paternity.

(d)That at the time the child is born, John Doe will formally acknowledge the paternity of said child.

(e)That Mary Roe will acknowledge that John Doe is the father of said child.

(f)That Mary Roe will consent to the adoption of said child by John Doe and Jane Doe.

"The agreement also provided that plaintiffs would pay Mary Roe the sum of $5,000 plus medical expenses. In addition, Mary Roe would be covered by sick leave, pregnancy disability insurance, and medical insurance from her employment while she is off work having the child and recuperating from the delivery.

"The plaintiffs allege that the disputed statutory provisions impermissibly infringe upon their constitutional right to privacy. This right, first recognized in *Griswold v. Connecticut*...was more recently described in *Carey v. Population Services International*.... In *Carey*, the Court specifically held that the decision 'whether or not to bear or beget a child' was among those protected by the constitutional right of privacy....

"While the decision to bear or beget a child has thus been found to be a fundamental interest protected by the right of privacy...we do not view this right as a valid prohibition to state interference in the plaintiffs' contractual arrangement. The statute in question does not directly prohibit John Doe and Mary Roe from having the child as planned. It acts instead to preclude plaintiffs from paying consideration in conjunction with their use of the state's adoption procedures. In effect, the plaintiffs' contractual agreement discloses a desire to use the adoption code to change the legal status of the child—i.e., its right to support, interstate succession, etc. We do not perceive this goal as within the realm of fundamental interests protected by the right to privacy from reasonable governmental regulation.

"The plaintiffs also allege that the state has no compelling interest sufficient to justify the prohibitions embodied in the disputed statutes and, in addition, that the provisions are drawn too wide to reflect any legitimate state interests in this area. Our disposition of the foregoing issue, however, renders consideration of this issue unnecessary.

"Affirmed."

DIAMOND V. CHAKRABARTY

(U.S. Supreme Court, 1980)
447 U.S. 303

May a live, human-made micro-organism be patented?

CHIEF JUSTICE BURGER:

* * *

"[I]n 1972, respondent Chakrabarty, a microbiologist, filed a patent application, assigned to the General Electric Company. The application asserted 36 claims related to Chakrabarty's invention of a 'a bacterium from the genus Pseudomonas containing therein at least two stable energy-generating plasmids, each of said plasmids providing a separate hydrocarbon degradative pathway.' This human-made, genetically engineered bacterium is capable of breaking down multiple components of crude oil. Because of this property, which is possessed by no naturally occurring bacteria, Chakrabarty's invention is believed to have significant value for the treatment of oil spills.

"Chakrabarty's patent claims were of three types: first, process claims for the method of producing the bacteria; second, claims for an inculum comprised of a carrier material floating on water, such as straw, and the new bacteria; and third, claims to the bacteria themselves. The patent examiner allowed the claims falling into the first two categories, but rejected claims for the bacteria. His decision rested on two grounds: (1) that micro-organisms are products of nature, and (2) that as living things they are not patentable subject matter....

* * *

"The Court of Customs and Patent Appeals, by a divided vote, reversed on the authority of its prior decision in *In re Bergy*,...which held 'the fact that micro-organisms...are alive...[is] without legal significance for purposes of the patent law....'

* * *

"To buttress its argument, the Government, with the support of *amicus*, points to grave risks that may be generated by research endeavors such as respondent's. The briefs present a gruesome parade of horribles. Scientists, among them Nobel laureates, are quoted suggesting that genetic research may pose a serious threat to the human race, or, at the very least, that the dangers are far too substantial to permit such research to proceed apace at this time. We are told that genetic research and related technological developments may spread pollution and disease, that it may result in a loss of genetic diversity, and that its practice may tend to depreciate the value of human life. These arguments are forcefully, even passionately presented; they remind us that, at times, human ingenuity seems unable to control fully the forces it creates — that, with Hamlet, it is sometimes better 'to bear those ills we have than fly to others that we know not of.'

"It is argued that this Court should weigh these potential hazards in considering whether respondent's invention is patentable subject matter...we disagree. The grant or denial of patents on micro-organisms is not likely to put an end to genetic research or to its attendant risks. The large amount of research that has already occurred when no researcher had sure knowledge that patent protection would be available suggests that legislative or judicial fiat as to patentability will not deter the scientific mind from probing into the unknown any more than Canute could determine the tides. Whether respondent's claims are patentable may determine whether research efforts are accelerated by the hope of reward or slowed by want of incentives, but that is all.

"What is more important is that we are without competence to entertain these arguments — either to brush them aside as fantasies generated by fear of the unknown, or to act on them. The choice we are urged to make is a matter of high policy for resolution within the legislative process after the kind of investigation, examination, and study that legislative bodies can provide and courts cannot. That process involves the balancing of competing values and interests, which in our democratic system is the business of elected representatives. Whatever their validity, the contentions now pressed on us should be addressed to the political branches of the government, the Congress and the Executive, and not to the Courts.

***

"Accordingly, the judgment of the Court of Customs and Patent Appeals is affirmed. Affirmed."

(Justice Brennan, White, Marshall, and Powell dissented.)

QUESTIONS

1. Should compulsory sterilization be used where criminal behavior has been shown to be genetically transferred? How high a probability of criminal trait transfer to offspring should be required for compulsory sterilization?
2. Should mentally retarded or physically defective persons be allowed to procreate? Suppose they would be able to care for their offspring? Suppose they would not be able to care for their offspring? Would it make any difference if the children were likely to be mentally retarded or physically defective?
3. How might religious values influence laws dealing with genetics and birth control? If religious values do influence these laws, would their constitutionality be brought into question?
4. Should government strictly regulate artificial insemination?
5. Does AID and surrogate motherhood challenge the foundations of marriage?
6. Should genetic screening be obligatory for the granting of a marriage license? For everyone? To obtain a job?
7. Is AID, genetic screening and surrogate motherhood a quest for the genetically perfect child?
8. Will the patenting of new life forms encourage dangerous experimentation with genetic material?

CHAPTER 3

THE PROBLEMS OF INFORMED CONSENT

INTRODUCTION

LACK of informed consent is, in a legal sense, battery. The tort principle of battery requires that persons control what happens to their body. Thus, to "touch" the body of one who has not assented is to subject oneself to possible liability. In order to protect oneself from liability, the medical professional must obtain the informed consent of the patient. That means the patient must be sufficiently informed about the proposed treatment.

The question of the meaning of "sufficient" information has divided American courts. Most courts hold that a physician must provide the information that a reasonable practitioner would provide who was in a similar community and who was from the same school of thought. Thus, this rule determines sufficiency by reference to established medical practices. A minority of courts require that information be provided that a reasonable man would think was material in considering whether to give consent to treatment. The "reasonable man" rule apparently has introduced greater uncertainty into the provision of informed consent and has made it more likely for patients to win malpractice suits.[1]

Both the rules recognize that certain risks may be so well known or so unlikely that they need not be disclosed. Both rules also recognize that in situations where the patient is in serious danger and unable to consent, informed consent is not required. Both rules also recognize the "therapeutic privilege," where doctors withhold information if it is judged to be in the best interests of the patients' health or welfare.[2]

Consent to medical treatment should, as a matter of law, be informed, voluntary, and competent. As a New York court noted in the early part of this century, "Every human being of adult years and sound mind has a right to determine what shall be done with

---

[1]Barber, Bernard: *Informed Consent in Medical Therapy and Research* (New Brunswick, Rutgers, 1980, pp. 35-41).
[2]Ibid., pp. 36-37.

his own body...."[3] There is also a strong tradition which emphasizes that patient welfare is best promoted by making the patient aware of what is to be done to him. In this way, the patient makes a choice of his treatment and is accountable for that decision.

However, consent does not always meet these goals. In an essay of remarkable candor, a physician has suggested that consent is far from informed, voluntary, and competent. Doctor E.G. Laforet wrote, "Few fabricated concepts of recent vintage have achieved the currency, uncritical and ungrudging, of 'informed consent.' The term is so semantically felicitous, so easy to say, so straightforward and uncomplicated, that it must seem churlish indeed to suggest that it is a fraud."[4]

What makes the goals of an informed, voluntary, and competent consent to medical treatment difficult to achieve? One problem is the great faith and trust many people have in physicians. Informed consent requires a questioning interaction between patient and physician. Rather than such a relationship, often the patient relates to the physician as a servant to a master. Thus, there is no interaction between the patient and the physician over the course of medical treatment. Instead of learning of options and risks associated with various procedures, the patient simply wilts before the master and exclaims, "Doctor, do whatever you think is best." It is a relationship between doctor and patient that is unfortunately frequently cultivated by physicians, perhaps in part because of a belief that the patient cannot best make a determination of the appropriate course of treatment. The master-servant relationship between physician and patient is also a far more simple and less-cumbersome relationship than that required by informed, voluntary, and competent consent.[5]

There is often a serious communications problem that makes informed consent difficult. One aspect of this problem is a lack of physician accessibility. Physicians may leave obtaining consent to subordinates, which makes it difficult for the patient to question the

---

[3]*Scholendorff v. New York Hospital,* 105 N.E. at 92-93 (1914).

[4]Quoted in Smith, Harmon L.:A valid consent—informed, voluntary, competent. In Robbins, Dennis A., and Dyer, Allen R. (Eds.):*Ethical Dimensions of Clinical Medicine* (Springfield, Thomas, 1981, p. 78). The complete article is Laforet, E.G. The fiction of informed consent (*Journal of the American Medical Association, 235*:1579-1585, 1976).

[5]See generally, Smith, op cit., pp. 70-81. The concern for informed consent by patients and the concern with the patient's rights in general is relatively new. See Veatch, Robert M.:*A Theory of Medical Ethics* (New York, Basic Books, 1981, pp. 47-49).

physician. Additionally, patients may feel that the physician has little time to spend with the patient and little time to be questioned by the patient about a medical procedure. When there is interaction between the physician and patient, informed consent can be limited by the different vocabularies of the physician and patient. Patients have been found to have a remarkable lack of knowledge of anatomy, medical terminology, and even routinely used words as "workup" and "history." However, physicians frequently persist in their use of the "special language of the hospital."[6]

Even if the patient and physician interact in an effort to produce informed consent, the problems of achieving consent that is informed, voluntary, and competent are immense. When a patient is desperately ill, it is difficult, and perhaps impossible, for that patient to rationally deliberate in order to calculate risks or alternative procedures. The patient may well grasp for any treatment that offers hope of recovery or promises a minimum of pain. Yet, such procedures may not be in the best interests of the patient. A hypothetical patient who is without pain, fear, or a sense of desperation might clearly see the irrationality of the actual patient's embrace of a questionable treatment, but it is the actual rather than hypothetical patient with whom physicians must deal.

The problems in obtaining an informed, voluntary, and competent consent are further complicated by those situations where the patient is a minor or is clearly incompetent. In the face of a patient's inability to consent, the consent of a third party is usually obtained. The assumption is that the third party (i.e. a court, a parent, or a spouse) can adequately represent the interests of the patient. These third parties, in effect, provide the consent on behalf of the patient. Much litigation surrounds this issue of informed consent for minors and incompetents.

---

[6]Barber, op cit., p. 88.

STRUNK V. STRUNK

(Court of Appeals of Kentucky, 1969)
445 S. W. 2d 145

May a kidney be removed for transplant purposes from an incompetent ward of the state so that the ward's brother may live?

JUDGE OSBORNE:

* * *

"...Tommy Strunk is twenty-eight years of age, married, an employee of the Penn State Railroad and a part-time student at the University of Cincinnati. Tommy is now suffering from chronic glomerulus nephritis, a fatal kidney disease. He is now being kept alive by frequent treatment on an artificial kidney, a procedure which cannot be continued much longer.

"Jerry Strunk is twenty-seven years of age, incompetent, and through proper legal proceedings has been committed to the Frankfort State Hospital and School, which is a state institution maintained for the feeble-minded. He has an IQ of approximately thirty-five, which corresponds with the mental age of approximately six years. He is further handicapped by a speech defect, which makes it difficult for him to communicate with persons who are not well acquainted with him. When it was determined that Tommy, in order to survive, would have to have a kidney, the doctors considered the possibility of using a kidney from a cadaver if and when one became available or one from a live donor if this could be made available. The entire family, his mother, father and a number of collateral relatives were tested. Because of incompatibility of blood type or tissue, none were medically acceptable as live donors. As a last resort, Jerry was tested and found to be highly acceptable....

"..A psychiatrist, in attendance to Jerry, who testified in the case, stated in his opinion the death of Tommy under these circumstances would have 'an extremely traumatic effect upon him' (Jerry).

"The Department of Mental Health of this Commonwealth has entered the case as *amicus curiae* and on the basis of its evaluation of the seriousness of the operation as opposed to the traumatic effect upon Jerry as a result of the loss of Tommy, recommended to the court that Jerry be permitted to undergo the surgery. Its recommendations are as follows:

> It is difficult for the mental defective to establish a firm sense of identity with another person and the acquisition of this necessary identity is dependent upon a person whom one can conveniently accept as a model and who at the same time is sufficiently flexible to allow the defective to detach himself with reassurances of continuity. His need to be social is not so much the necessity of a formal and mechanical contact with other human beings as it is the necessity of a close intimacy with other men, the desirability of a real community of feeling, and urgent need for a unity of understanding. Purely mechanical and formal contact with other men does not offer any treatment for the behavior of a mental defective; only those who are able to communicate intimately are of value to hospital treatment in these cases. And this generally is a member of the family.
>
> In view of this knowledge, we now have particular interest in this case. Jerry Strunk, a mental defective, has emotions and reactions on a scale comparable to that of a normal person. He identifies with his brother Tom; Tom is his model, his tie with his family. Tom's life is vital to the continuity of Jerry's improvement at Frankfort State Hospital and School. The testimony of the hospital representative reflected the importance to Jerry of his visits with his family and the constant inquiries Jerry made about Tom's coming to see him. Jerry is aware he plays a role in the relief of this tension. We the Department of Mental Health must take all possible steps to prevent the occurrence of any guilt feelings Jerry would have if Tom were to die.
>
> The necessity of Tom's life to Jerry's treatment and eventual rehabilitation is clearer in view of the fact that Tom is his only living sibling and at the death of their parents, now in their fifties, Jerry will have no concerned, intimate communication so necessary to his stability and optimal functioning.
>
> The evidence shows that at the present level of medical knowledge, it is quite remote that Tom would be able to survive several cadaver transplants. Tom has a much better chance of survival if the kidney transplant from Jerry takes place.

"Upon this appeal we are faced with the fact that all members of the immediate family have recommended the transplant. The Department of Mental Health has likewise made its recommendation. The county court has given its approval. The circuit court has found that it would be to the best interest of the ward of the state that the procedure be carried out. Throughout the legal proceedings, Jerry has been represented by a guardian *ad litem*, who has continually questioned the power of the state to authorize the removal of an organ from the body of an incompetent who is a ward of the state. We are full cognizant of the fact that the question before us is unique. Insofar as we have been able to learn, no similar set of facts has come before the highest court of any of the states of this nation or the federal courts....

"The medical practice of transferring tissue from one part of the human body to another (autografting) and from one human being to another (homografting) is rapidly becoming a common clinical practice. In many cases the transplants take as well where the tissue is dead as when it is alive. This has made practicable the establishment of tissue banks where such material can be stored for future use. Vascularized grafts of lungs, kidneys, and hearts are becoming increasingly common. These grafts must be of functioning, living cells with blood vessels remaining anatomically intact. The chance of success in the transfer of these organs is greatly increased when the donor and the donee are genetically related....

"The renal transplant is becoming the most common of the organ transplants. This is because the normal body has two functioning kidneys, one of which it can reasonably do without, thereby making it possible for one person to donate a kidney to another. Testimony in this record shows that there have been over 2500 kidney transplants performed in the United States up to this date. The process can be effected under present techniques with minimal danger to both the donor and the donee. Doctors Hamburger and Crosneir describe the risk to the donor as follows: '...The immediate operative risk of unilateral nephrectomy in a healthy subject has been calculated as approximately 0.05 percent. The long-term risk is more difficult to estimate, since the various types of renal disease do not appear to be more frequent or more severe in individuals with solitary kidneys than in normal subjects. On the other hand, the development of surgical problems, trauma, or neoplasms, with the possible necessity of nephrectomy, do increase the long-term risks in living donors; the long-term risk, on this basis, has been estimated at 0.07 percent....'*

* * *

"We are of the opinion that a chancery court does have sufficient inherent power to authorize the operation. The circuit court having

---

*Hamburger and Crosneir, Moral and ethical problems in transplantation. In Rapaport and Dausset (Eds.): *Human Transplantation*, *37*, 1968.

found that the operative procedures in this instance are to the best interest of Jerry Strunk and this finding having been based upon substantial evidence, we are of the opinion the judgment should be affirmed...."

* * *

(Hill, C.J., Milliken and Reed, J.J., concur.)

STEINFELD, JUDGE, DISSENTING:

"Apparently because of my indelible recollection of a government which, to the everlasting shame of its citizens, embarked on a program of genocide and experimentation with human bodies, I have been more troubled in reaching a decision in this case than in any other. My sympathies and emotions are torn between a compassion to aid an ailing young man and a duty to fully protect unfortunate members of society.

"...Courts have restricted the activities of the committee to that which is for the best interest of the incompetent.... The wishes of the members of the family or the desires of the guardian to be helpful to the apparent objects of the ward's bounty have not been a criterion....

* * *

"...The majority opinion is predicated upon the finding of the circuit court that there will be psychological benefits to the ward but point out that the incompetent has the mentality of a six-year-old child. It is common knowledge beyond dispute that the loss of a close relative or a friend to a six-year-old child is not a major impact. Opinions concerning psychological trauma are at best most nebulous. Furthermore, there are no guarantees that the transplant will become a surgical success, it being well known that body rejection of transplanted organs is frequent. The life of the incompetent is not in danger, but the surgical procedure advocated creates some peril.

* * *

"Unquestionably, the attitudes and attempts of the committee and members of the family of the two young men whose critical problems now confront us are commendable, natural, and beyond reproach. However, they refer us to nothing indicating that they are privileged to authorize the removal of one of the kidneys of the incompetent for the purpose of donation, and they cite no statutory or other authority vesting such right in the courts. The proof shows that less compatible donors are available and that the kidney of a cadaver could be used, although the odds of operational success are not as great in such case as they would be with the fully compatible donor brother.

"I am unwilling to hold that the gates should be open to permit the removal of an organ from an incompetent for transplant, at least until such time as it is conclusively demonstrated that it will be of significant benefit to the incompetent....

"Neikirk and Palmore, J.J., join with me in this dissent."

* * *

HART V. BROWN

(Connecticut Superior Court, 1972)
289 A. 2d 386

May parents of identical twins consent to transplantation of a kidney from one twin to the other? The twins were seven years and ten months old. A transplant was necessary to save the life of one twin. The child had had both of her kidneys removed. Given the child's age, dialysis was viewed as risky. There was a fifty-fifty chance the child would live five years if dialysis was used. The other twin was considered an ideal donor. Prognosis for good health and long life was good for both twins if the transplant was performed.

JUDGE TESTO:

* * *

"Since 1966, it is reported in the Ninth Report of the *Human Renal Transplant Registry*, twelve twin grafts have been performed. All twelve have been successful, as reported by the *Registry*, at one- and two-year follow-ups. In the identical twin donations since 1966, grafts are functioning at 100 percent. Before 1955, because of technical matters, the survival rate was about 90 percent. Of all isografts followed since 1966, all are successful. In this type of a graft there is substantially a 100 percent chance that the twins will live out a normal life span — emotionally and physically.

"If a parent donates the kidney, the statistics show less success. The average percent of success in that type of transplant has been 70 percent at one year and 65 percent or so over a two-year period. The falloff thereafter runs another 5 to 10 more percent per year.

The long-range survival of a parent transplant runs around 50 to 55 percent over a period of five years and appears to fall off to about 37 percent over a period of seven years.

"The side effects of the immunosuppressive drugs in a parental homograft are numerous and include the possibility of bone marrow toxicity, liver damage, and a syndrome called Cushing syndrome — a roundish face, a 'buffalo hump' on the back of the neck, and growth retardation. It has also been reported that two suicides have occurred because of the psychological effect upon young girls resulting from immunosuppressive drugs. An overall percentage of around 70 to 77 percent would be expected to survive two years from a parental graft. It is also possible that 40 to 50 percent of the patients might still be surviving at near ten years with a parental graft.

"Of 3000 recorded kidney operations of live donors, there is reported only one death of a donor, and even this death may have been from causes unrelated to the procedure. The short-range risk to a donor is negligible. The operating surgeon testified that the surgical risk is no more than the risk of the anesthesia. The operative procedure would last about two-and-one-half hours. There would be some minor postoperative pain but no more than in any other surgical procedure. The donor would be hospitalized for about eight days and would be able to resume normal activities in thirty days. Assuming an uneventful recovery, the donor would thereafter be restricted only from violent contact sports. She would be able to engage in all of the normal life activities of an active young girl. Medical testimony indicated that the risk to the donor is such that life insurance actuaries do not rate such individuals higher than those with two kidneys. The only real risk would be trauma to the one remaining kidney, but testimony indicated that such trauma is extremely rare in civilian life.

***

"A psychiatrist who examined the donor gave testimony that the donor has a strong identification with her twin sister. He also testified that if the expected successful results are achieved they would be of immense benefit to the donor in that the donor would be better off in a family that was happy than in a family that was distressed and in that it would be a very great loss to the donor if the donee were to die from her illness.

"The donor has been informed of the operation and insofar as she may be capable of understanding she desires to donate her kidney so that her sister may return to her. A clergyman was also a witness and his testimony was that the decision by the parents of the donor and donee was morally and ethically sound. The court-appointed guardian *ad litem* for the donor gave testimony that he conferred with the parents, the physicians, the donor, and other men in the religious profession, and he has consented to the performance of the operation.

***

"The court understands that the operation on the donee is a necessity for her continued life; that there are negligible risks involved to both donor and donee; that to subject the donee to a parental homograft may be cruel and inhuman because of the possible side effects to the immunosuppressive drugs; that the prognosis for good health and long life to both children is excellent; that there is no known opposition to having the operation performed; that it will be most beneficial to the donee; and that it will be of some benefit to the donor. To prohibit the natural parents and the guardians *ad litem* of the minor children the right to give their consent under these circumstances, where there is supervision by this court and other persons in examining their judgment, would be most unjust, inequitable and injudicious. Therefore, natural parents of a minor should have the right to give their consent to an isograft kidney transplantation procedure when their motivation and reasoning are favorably reviewed by a community representation which includes a court of equity."

***

IN RE ROTKOWITZ

(Domestic Relations Court of City of New York, 1941)
25 N.Y.S. 2d 624

May a court order surgery on a ten-year-old child for a non-life-threatening defect?

JUSTICE PANKEN:

* * *

"...A child who is deprived of the use of its limb which becomes progressively worse cannot have a sense of security.... It cannot take its proper place in the group in which it lives. To the extent that medical science can correct the deformity or the limitation of the use of a limb, that service should be accorded.

"When the Legislature clothed this court with the power to make an order for surgical care, it cannot be said that an order is to be made only in a case where the parents consented to such order. I must conclude that it was the intention of the Legislature to give power to the Justices of this Court to order an operation not only in an instance where the life of the child is to be saved but also in instances where the health, the limb, the person or the future of the child is at stake.

"The report submitted by the New York Orthopedic Hospital specifically states that an operation is necessary to correct the deformity of the right lower extremity from which the child is suffering and which is becoming aggravated. The deformity was induced by poliomyelitis. This operation, the doctor testified, is not a serious one; it is absolutely necessary to stabilize the foot and prevent aggravation and extention of the deformity.

"This surgery was advised four years ago when the child was first examined. It appeared to be necessary then. The condition has become worse. The operation was not performed because of the opposition of the father.

"Doctor Frank J. Tarsney, a duly licensed physician and a specialist in orthopedics, testified that he had examined this child in November of 1940, and at that time found that an operation was necessary to prevent further deformity and immobility and for correction of the condition existing. I asked him to re-examine the child on the day the hearing was had before me, to wit, the 28th of February, 1941. Less than four months elapsed since his first examination. His testimony is that the condition has become aggravated and the deformity is more pronounced. He testified that the condition will become worse as time goes by unless operative correction is had now....

"The father of the child testified and said, insofar as it was possible for him to make himself articulate, that he was opposed to the operation. He gave no reason why he is opposed. The mother testified that she is very anxious that the child be operated on. The situation is that one parent is in favor of the operation; the other opposed. The one who has the intelligence to be concerned about the future of the child wants the operation; the other who is either unconcerned or has no capacity to be concerned is opposed to it. That creates a situation almost parallel to the two women, each of whom claimed to be the mother of a child, and when King Solomon said he would give each half of the child, the true mother was ready to give the whole child to the one who was not the mother.

"...The hospital authorities refuse to perform the operation without the consent of both parents, unless ordered by the Court.

"The question before this Court is whether an order should be made for such operation. It is my opinion that the best interests of the child now and for the future require an order to be made regardless of the opposition of the father. Such an order would be permissive in face of opposition of both parents."

* * *

IN RE SEIFERTH

(Court of Appeals of New York, 1955)
127 N.E. 2d 820

May a child be forced to undergo non-life saving surgery against his wishes and the wishes of the child's father?

JUDGE VAN VOORHIS:

"This is a case involving a fourteen-year-old boy with cleft palate and harelip, whose father holds strong convictions with which the boy has become imbued against medicine and surgery. This proceeding has been instituted by the deputy commissioner of the Erie County Health Department on petition to the Children's Court to have Martin declared a neglected child, and to have his custody transferred from his parents to the commissioner of Social Welfare of Erie County for the purpose of consenting to such medical, surgical and dental services as may be necessary to rectify his condition. The medical testimony is to the effect that such cases are almost always given surgical treatment at an earlier age, and the older the patient is, the less favorable are likely to be the results, according to experience. The surgery recommended by the plastic surgeon called for petitioner consists of three operations: (1) repair of the harelip by bringing the split together; (2) closing the cleft or split in the rear of the palate, the boy being already too late in life to have the front part mended by surgery; and (3) repairing the front part of the palate by dental appliances. The only risk of mortality is the negligible one due to the use of anesthesia....

"Even after the operation, Martin will not be able to talk normally, at least not without going to a school for an extended period for concentrated speech therapy. There are certain phases of a child's life when the importance of these defects becomes of greater significance....

***

"The father testified that 'If the child decides on an operation, I shall not be opposed,' and that 'I want to say in a few years the child should decide for himself...whether to have the operation or not.' The father believes in mental healing by letting 'the forces of the universe work on the body,' although he denied that this is an established religion of any kind.... There is no doubt, however, that the father is strong minded about this, and has inculcated a distrust and dread of surgery in the boy since childhood.

***

"On February 11, 1954, Martin, his father and attorney met...in Judge Wylegala's chambers. Judge Wylegala wrote in his opinion that Martin '...had come to the conclusion that he should try for some time longer to close the cleft palate and the split lip himself through 'natural forces.'" After stating that an order for surgery would have been granted without hesitation if this proceeding had been instituted before this child acquired convictions of his own, Judge Wylegala summed up his conclusions as follows: 'After duly deliberating upon the psychological effect of surgery upon this mature, intelligent boy, schooled as he had been for all of his young years in the existence of 'forces of nature' and his fear of surgery upon the human body, I have come to the conclusion that no order should be made at this time compelling the child to submit to surgery. His condition is not emergent and there is no serious threat to his health or life. He has time until he becomes 21 years of age to apply for financial assistance under County and State aid to physically handicapped children to have the corrections made....' The petition accordingly was dismissed.

"The Appellate Division, Fourth Department, reversed by a divided court, and granted the petition requiring Martin Seiferth to submit to surgery.

"As everyone agrees, there are important considerations both ways. The Children's Court has power in drastic situations to direct the operation over the objection of parents.... Nevertheless, there is no present emergency, time is less of the essence than it was a few years ago insofar as concerns the physical prognosis, and we are impressed by the circumstance that in order to benefit from the operation upon the cleft palate, it will almost certainly be necessary to enlist Martin's cooperation in developing normal speech patterns through a lengthy course in concentrated speech therapy. It will be almost impossible to secure his cooperation if he continued to believe, as he does now, that it will be necessary 'to remedy the surgeon's distortion first and then go back to the primary task of healing the body.' This is an aspect of the problem with which petitioner's plastic surgeon did not especially concern himself, for he did not attempt to view the case from the psychological viewpoint of this misguided youth. Upon the other hand, the Children's Court Judge, who saw and heard the witnesses, and arranged the conferences for the boy and his father...appears to have been keenly aware of this aspect of the situation, and to have concluded that less would be lost by permitting the lapse of several more years, when the boy may make his own decision to submit to plastic surgery, than might be sacrificed if he were compelled to undergo it now against his sincere and frightened antagonism....

"The order of the Appellate Division should be reversed and that of the Children's Court reinstated...."

JUDGE FULD, JOINED BY JUDGE DESMOND AND JUDGE BURKE, DISSENTING:

"Every child has a right, so far as is possible, to lead a normal life and, if his parents, through viciousness or ignorance, act in such a way as to endanger that right, the courts should, as the legislature has provided, act on his behalf....

* * *

"...Whether the child condones the neglect, whether he is willing to let his parents do as they choose, surely cannot be operative on the question as to whether or not they are guilty of neglect. They are not interested or concerned with whether he does or does not want the essential operation. They have arbitrarily taken the position that there is to be no surgery. What these parents are doing, by their failure to provide for an operation, however well-intentioned, is far worse than beating this child or denying him food or clothing. To the boy, and his future, it makes no difference that it may be ignorance rather than viciousness that will perpetuate his unfortunate condition. If parents are actually mistreating or neglecting a child, the circumstance that he may not mind it cannot alter the fact that they are guilty of neglect and it cannot render their conduct permissible.

"The welfare and interests of a child are at stake. A court should not place upon his shoulders one of the most momentous and far-reaching decisions of his life. The court should make the decision, as the statute contemplates, and leave to the good sense and sound judgment of the public authorities the job of preparing the boy for the operation and of getting him as adjusted to it as possible. We should not put off decision in the hope and on the chance that the child may change his mind and submit at some future time to the operation."

* * *

RUBY V. MASSEY

(U.S. District Court, 1978)
452 F. Supp. 361

Parents challenged the refusal of hospitals to perform sterilizations upon their severely mentally retarded and physically handicapped daughters.

BLUMENFELD, JUDGE:

* * *

"...Plaintiffs request an injunction ordering the defendant University of Connecticut Health center and named physicians employed by the Center to 'refrain from refusing' to perform surgical hysterectomies on their three non-institutionalized mentally re-tarded children and a declaratory judgment that the defendants' failure to perform the hysterectomies is unconstitutional as a violation of their right to privacy, to equal protection of the laws, and to due process of law.

"The three girls (Susan, aged 12; Valerie, aged 13; and Lynn,· aged 15) are severely mentally retarded and physically handicapped (blind-deaf). Susan and Valerie have no useful communication abilities; Lynn has only minimal ability to communicate. Although at present the girls are residents of a special school during the week and live with their parents on the weekends, custodial care is inevitable for each of them because of their grossly impaired mental functioning and physical handicaps. The Diamonds have sought Valerie's admission to one of the two state institutions for the retarded since 1968. Priscilla Pearl has sought Lynn's admission since 1970. Neither girl is apt to be admitted to a state institution in the foreseeable future.

"Each of the girls shows signs of sexual development....

"The girls are presumably capable of conceiving, but if they were to become pregnant, they would be subject to grave risks because they are incapable of communicating with a physician about their own physical condition...the girls cannot be examined internally or tested...without being put under a general anesthetic each time, with all the dangers posed by that process.

"The plaintiffs have consulted with a number of physicians and social workers who have concluded that therapeutic uterectomies (sterilizations) are 'medically indicated.' The defendants' agent, Doctor Osborne, agrees that the sterilizations are 'medically indicated.' He is professionally qualified to perform the surgery and he is willing to do so.

"...The defendants have stipulated that their refusal 'is based solely upon their legal counsel's judgment that the plaintiff parents' consent to have such surgery performed...is not now or may not be in the future legally sufficient to protect the Health Center against possible civil liability.' This concern is apparently widespread among the Connecticut hospitals, for the plaintiffs unsuccessfully sought to have the sterilizations performed at several other (private) hospitals in the state before bringing the instant action.

"Two factors are said to account for the hospitals' fear of civil liability. First, there is no statute which expressly empowers parents and/or guardians of retarded persons to give legally sufficient consent to such sterilizations; and second, there is no Connecticut statute which expressly authorizes the sterilization of mentally incompetent persons in general (private) hospitals.

"It will be helpful to distinguish between two discrete claims made by the parents: (1) that their right as parents to familial privacy entitles them to give legally sufficient consent to the sterilization of their daughters; and (2) that their daughters are entitled to the benefits of Conn. Gen. Stat. section 19-569g, which does provide for sterilization of inmates of certain state institutions. The statute...allows the institutions' superintendents to submit the sterilization question to a board of doctors, and then to apply to a probate court for judicial authorization to perform the operations....

"When a parent decides to call a physician to care for her child, she may give lawful consent for him to administer that medical or surgical treatment which, in the doctor's professional opinion, is necessary or advisable for the health of her child. The parents' authority in their own household to direct the rearing of their children has a constitutional underpinning. The Supreme Court has said: 'It is cardinal with us that the custody, care and nurture of the child reside first in the parents, whose primary function and freedom include preparation for obligations the state can neither support nor hinder....' But this case is not concerned with the general support of medical services for a child to which her parent may consent, nor with the correlative duty upon the parent to provide them for her minor children.

"Because surgical sterilization has an immediate effect, both upon the health of a patient and upon her ability to procreate, it impinges upon two separate interests. There is '...an important and legitimate interest in preserving and protecting the health of the pregnant woman...and...another important and legitimate interest in protecting the potentiality of human life. These interests are separate and distinct....'

"So much has already been written to support the numerous decisions of the Supreme Court holding that a decision whether to bear or beget a child merits special constitutional protection, that it would be redundant to repeat it here....

* * *

"However, in this long line of cases which undeviatingly hold that the Constitution protects the freedom of even an immature teenager to decide for herself whether to bear or beget a child, no case has considered the question of who may make the sterilization decision for the child who is mentally incapable of deciding for herself. The fact that in this case the parents seek to have the children's rights exercised in favor of sterilization, rather than against it, does not affect the character of the right. They may neither veto nor give valid consent to the sterilization of their children.

* * *

"This lawsuit is unmistakably a poignant cry for help from these children uttered in their behalf by their parents. These children are what they are; they are unable to come to terms in reality sufficiently to make the decisions which are only theirs to make. That they are incapable of comprehending the consequences of their actions is clear beyond question. The fact that the demand for an 'informed' decision from each of the children is an impossible one to meet makes imperative the need for an authoritative decision on their behalf.

"...Although Connecticut's law does not completely ignore the problem of a mentally incompetent minor's inability to give consent to a sterilization operation, it does not in terms specifically apply to the situation of the plaintiffs in this case because their children are not inmates of either the Mansfield or Southbury Training Schools.

* * *

"The question then is whether it is a violation of the constitutional right of the plaintiffs to equal protection of the laws to deny them access to the method for obtaining valid consent to a sterilization operation as provided for in section 19-569g.

* * *

"Whether the plaintiffs have been denied access to the court in violation of the equal protection clause of the Fourteenth Amendment depends upon two factors. First, the interest which the plaintiffs seek to protect must be 'fundamental.' Second, the action of a court of law must be objectively necessary to protect that interest.

If both of these are present, it is a violation of equal protection to deny them access to the court.... The monopolization of access is clearly present in this case since a 'judicial proceeding [is] the only effective means for resolving the dispute at hand....' What has been shown earlier in this opinion is more than ample to demonstrate that the right of the plaintiff's children to be sterilized is 'fundamental' because it is rooted in the Constitution. And, in view of the fact that no one may subject them to a sterilization operation without their consent, 'resort to the state courts is the only avenue,' ...to obtain valid consent for such operations. It is both subjectively and objectively impossible for valid consent of these plaintiffs' children to be otherwise obtained.

"The reasons advanced by the defendants in their brief to justify the state for treating residents in its two institutions differently from all other mentally incompetent children are: 'Once institutionalized the state is responsible for the care of these individuals. To avoid problems of undesired pregnancy the state may rationally decide to sterilize some individuals. State officials might otherwise be subjected to liability for improper supervision if an institutionalized woman were to become pregnant. Some of the patients within the institution are wards of the state. Should one give birth, the state would be burdened by the additional expense of raising a child.'

"The interests which the state asserts may well justify it in establishing a method for obtaining authority to perform sterilization operations on its wards. The state is simply discharging a parental obligation. None of these interests will be jeopardized if the same statutory process is made available to those incompetent children who have not been institutionalized. If the state may rationally decide to sterilize some individuals to avoid incomprehensible pregnancy, it makes shamefully limited sense to contend that the same right should be denied to others in the same situation.

"...Exclusion of plaintiffs from the benefits of the statute is not necessary to further the state's interest; it is not even relevant. Denying to the plaintiffs as guardians the right the state has created for itself as guardian invidiously discriminates against the plaintiffs' children with respect to their fundamental interest in privacy. No matter what legal standard is used to test the state's refusal to permit the plaintiffs access to its method for obtaining consent, the defendants have not shown the justification which the equal protection clause requires for monopolizing the process for obtaining valid consent to a sterilization operation....

* * *

"Accordingly, it is the order of this court that the defendants are enjoined from refusing to provide the plaintiffs with services identical to those provided to inmates of the Mansfield Training School and the Southbury Training School to enable them to obtain consent of a probate court to the sterilization operations upon them."

* * *

RELF V. WEINBERGER

(U.S. District Court, 1974)
372 F. Supp. 1196

The plaintiffs challenged federal regulations providing for federally funded sterilizations.

GESELL, DISTRICT JUDGE:

* * *

"Congress has authorized the funding of a full range of family planning services under two basic procedures. The Public Health Service administers federal grants to state health agencies and to public and private projects for the provision of family planning services to the poor...and the Social and Rehabilitation Service provides funds for such services under the Medicaid and Aid to Families of Dependent Children programs....

"Although there is no specific reference to sterilization in any of the family planning statutes nor in the legislative history surrounding their passage, the Secretary has considered sterilization to fall within the general statutory scheme, and Congress has been made aware of this position. But until recently, there were no particular rules or regulations governing the circumstances under which sterilizations could be funded under these statutes.

"Sterilization of females or males is irreversible. The total number of these sterilizations is clearly of national significance. Few realize that over 16 percent of the married couples in this country between the ages of 20 and 39 have had a sterilization operation. Over the last few years, an estimated 100,000 to 150,000 low-income persons have been sterilized annually under federally funded programs. Virtually all of these people have been adults; only about 2,000 to 3,000 per year have been under 21 years of age and fewer than 300 have been under 18. There are no statistics in the record indicating what percentage of these patients were mentally incompetent.

"Although Congress has been insistent that all family planning programs function on a purely voluntary basis, there is uncontroverted evidence in the record that minors and other incompetents have been sterilized with federal funds and that an indefinite number of poor people have been improperly coerced into accepting a sterilization operation under the threat that various federally supported welfare benefits would be withdrawn unless they submitted to irreversible sterilization. Patients receiving Medicaid assistance at childbirth are evidently the most frequent targets of this pressure, as the experiences of plaintiffs Waters and Walker illustrate. Mrs. Waters was actually refused medical assistance by her attending physician unless she submitted to a tubal ligation after the birth. Other examples were documented.

"When such deplorable incidents began to receive nationwide public attention...the Secretary took steps to restrict the circumstances under which recipients of federal family planning funds could conduct sterilization operations....

***

"...Briefly, they are as follows:

(1) Legally competent adults must give their 'informed consent' to sterilization. Such consent must be evidenced by a written and signed document indicating, *inter alia*, that the patient is aware of the benefits and costs of sterilization and of the fact that he may withdraw from the operation without losing federal benefits....

(2) Legally competent persons under the age of 18 must also give such written consent. In these situations, a special Review Committee of independent persons from the community must also have determined that the proposed sterilization is in the best interest of the patient, taking into consideration (a) the expected mental and physical impact of pregnancy and motherhood on the patient, if female, or the expected mental impact of fatherhood, if male, and (b) the expected immediate and long-term mental and physical impact of sterilization on the patient.... The Review Committee must also (a)

review appropriate medical, social and psychological information concerning the patient, including the age of the patient, alternative family planning methods, and the adequacy of consent, and (b) interview the patient, both parents of the patient (if available), and such other persons as in its judgment will contribute pertinent information....

(3) Legally incompetent minors must be afforded the above safeguards, and, in addition, a state court of competent jurisdiction must determine that the proposed sterilization is in the best interest of the patient....

(4) The sterilization of mental incompetents of all ages must also be sanctioned by a Review Committee and a court. However, personal consent is not required — it is enough that the patient's 'representative' requests sterilization.... Although defendants interpret the term 'representative' to mean a person empowered under state law to consent to the sterilization on behalf of the patient, no such definition appears in the regulations themselves.

"Plaintiffs do not oppose the voluntary sterilization of poor persons under federally funded programs. However, they contend that these regulations are both illegal and arbitrary because they authorize *involuntary* sterilizations without statutory justification. They argue forcefully that sterilization of minors or mental incompetents is necessarily involuntary in the nature of things. Further, they claim that sterilization of competent adults under these regulations can be undertaken without insuring the request for sterilization is in actuality voluntary. The Secretary defends the regulations and insists that only 'voluntary' sterilization is permitted under their terms.

***

"For the reasons developed below, the Court finds that the Secretary has no statutory authority under the family planning sections of the Social Security or Public Health Services acts to fund the sterilization of any person incompetent under state law to consent to such an operation, whether because of minority or mental deficiency. It also finds that the challenged regulations are arbitrary and unreasonable in that they fail to implement the congressional command that federal family planning funds not be used to coerce indigent patients into submitting to sterilization. In short, federally assisted family planning sterilizations are permissible only with the voluntary, knowing and uncoerced consent of individuals competent to give such consent. This result requires an injunction against substantial portions of the proposed regulations and their revision to insure that all sterilizations funded under the family planning sections are voluntary in the full sense of that term and that sterilization of incompetent minors and adults is prevented.

"...The Secretary argues that...Congress intended that minors personally and incompetents through their representatives would be able to consent to sterilization.... That conclusion is unwarranted.

"Although the term 'voluntary' is nowhere defined in the statutes under consideration, it is frequently encountered in the law. Even its dictionary definition assumes an exercise of free will and clearly precludes the existence of coercion or force.... And its use in the statutory and decisional law, at least when important human rights are at stake, entails a requirement that the individual have at his disposal the information necessary to make his decision and the mental competence to appreciate the significance of that information....

"No person who is mentally incompetent can meet these standards, nor can the consent of a representative, however sufficient under state law, impute voluntariness to the individual actually undergoing irreversible sterilization. Minors would also appear to lack the knowledge, maturity and judgment to satisfy these standards with regard to such an important issue, whatever may be their competence to rely on devices or medication that temporarily frustrates procreation. This is the reasoning that provides the basis for nearly universal common law and statutory rule that minors and mental incompetents cannot consent to medical operations....

"The statutory references to minors and mental incompetents do not contradict this conclusion, for they appear only in the context of family planning services in general. Minors, for example, are not legally incompetent for all purposes, and many girls of child-bearing age are undoubtedly sufficiently aware of the relevant considerations to use temporary contraceptives that intrude far less on fundamental rights. However, the Secretary has not demonstrated and the Court cannot find that Congress deemed such children capable of voluntarily consenting to an irreversible operation involving the basic human right to procreate. Nor can the Court find in the face of repeated warnings concerning voluntariness, that Congress authorized the imposition of such a serious deprivation upon mental incompetents at the will of an unspecified 'representative.'

"The regulations also fail to provide the procedural safeguards necessary to insure that even competent adults voluntarily request sterilization. Plaintiffs would require an elaborate hearing process prior to the operation to remedy this problem. The Secretary, however, has determined that the consent document procedure set forth in the existing regulations is adequate in most instances to insure a knowledgeable decision, and the Court finds that this determination is not unreasonable. In one respect, however, the consent procedure must be improved. Even a fully informed individual cannot make a 'voluntary' decision concerning sterilization if he has been subjected to coercion from doctors or project officers. Despite specific statutory language forbidding the recipients of federal family planning funds to threaten a cutoff of program benefits unless the individual submits to sterilization and despite clear evidence that such coercion is actually being applied, the challenged regulations contain no clear safeguard against this abuse. Although the required consent document must state that the patient can withdraw his consent to sterilization without losing other program benefits, there is nothing to prohibit the use of such coercion to extract the initial consent.

"In order to prevent express or implied threats, which would obviate the Secretary's entire framework of procedural safeguards, and to insure compliance with the statutory language, the Court concludes that the regulations must also be amended to require that individuals seeking sterilization be orally informed at the very outset that no federal benefits can be withdrawn because of a failure to accept sterilization. This guarantee must also appear prominently at the top of the consent document already required by the regulations. To permit sterilization without this essential safeguard is an unreasonable and arbitrary interpretation of the congressional mandate.

* * *

"This controversy has arisen during a period of rapid change in the field of birth control. In recent years, through the efforts of dedicated proponents of family planning, birth-control information and services have become widely available. Aided by the growing acceptance of family planning, medical science has steadily improved and diversified the techniques of birth prevention and control. Advancements in artificial insemination and in the understanding of genetic attributes are also affecting the decision to bear children. There are even suggestions in the scientific literature that the sex of the children may soon be subject to parental control. And over this entire area lies the spector of overpopulation, with its possible impact upon the food supply, interpersonal relations, privacy, and the enjoyment of our 'inalienable rights.'

"Surely the Federal Government must move cautiously in this area, under well-defined policies determined by Congress after full consideration of constitutional and far-reaching social implications. The dividing line between family planning and eugenics is murky. And yet the Secretary, through the regulations at issue, seeks to sanction one of the most drastic methods of population control — the involuntary irreversible sterilization of men and women — without any legislative guidance. Whatever might be the merits of limiting irresponsible reproduction, which each year places increasing numbers of unwanted or mentally defective children into tax-supported institutions, it is for Congress and not individual social workers and physicians to determine the manner in which federal funds should be used to support such a program. We should not drift into a policy which has unfathomed implications and which permanently deprives unwilling or immature citizens of their ability to procreate without adequate legal safeguards and a legislative determination of the appropriate standards in light of the general welfare and individual rights."

***

KARP V. COOLEY

(U.S. District Court, 1972)
349 F. Supp. 827

This issue of informed consent when using new and revolutionary medical techniques was encountered when Mr. Haskell Karp underwent surgery to replace his heart with a mechanical heart.

JUDGE SINGLETON:

***

"...Upon admission, Mr. Karp signed...an authorization for medical and/or surgical treatment which reads: 'I hereby authorize the physician or physicians in charge of Haskell (None) Karp to administer any treatment; or to administer such anesthetics; and perform such operations as may be deemed necessary or advisable in the diagnosis and treatment of this patient....' Mr. Karp remained as a patient in the hospital for several weeks being examined and treated by several doctors associated with the hospital. During this period of time, Doctor Cooley suggested that Mr. Karp's desire for a more active and productive life-style could best be achieved by a heart transplant. Mr. Karp rejected his suggestion and preferred to undergo ventriculoplasty surgery (wedge procedure) which Doctor Cooley had developed.... This surgery necessitates the excision of part of the diseased tissues in the left ventricle in order that the remaining tissue and heart muscle can function at its optimal level.

"As regards the informed — consent issue, Doctor Cooley testified that he discussed various aspects of the surgery in question with Mr. Karp on at least three occasions: once the week before April 4, again at 10:30 p.m. on the night of April 2 and a brief chat on April 3. According to Doctor Cooley's testimony, of these the most significant was that of April 2. On that occasion, Doctor Cooley explained to Mr. Karp that the ventriculoplasty surgery could be performed on Friday, April 4, 1969. Doctor Cooley testified he explained the risks, grave dangers and backup procedures involved therein. Further, he explained to Mr. Karp that there was a "70-30" chance of his surviving the ventriculoplasty operation. Doctor Cooley explained, as was stated in the written consent form, that if death appeared imminent, that his heart would be removed and a mechanical heart substitute (sometimes referred to as the Cooley-Liotta mechanical heart) inserted. Doctor Cooley testified that he told Mr. Karp the mechanical heart substitute would not be permanent but would be replaced as soon as possible by a human heart transplant, but that at that time there was no heart donor available, nor any prospect of one. Doctor Cooley also testified that he promised Mr. Karp he would do all that is humanly possible to insure his well-being and improve his patient's, that is, Mr. Karp, condition. At that time, Mr. Karp gave him his verbal consent to the surgery.

"Mrs. Karp testified that if Doctor Cooley did see her husband that evening (April 2, 1969) that it would have to have been very late, for she usually stayed until after 10:00 p.m. with her husband.

However, she also testified that on the night in question she went out to dinner at a friend's home late in the evening and did not return to the hospital that night until after his dinner and visit.

"Rabbi Wilkin, a Jewish chaplain for the medical center who had been calling on Mr. Karp daily since his admission to the hospital, testified that on one of the days during the week of surgery (week beginning Monday, March 31, 1969), Mr. Karp had an urgent message sent to him to come to his room. The Rabbi went to his room, where he found Mr. Karp alone. Mr. Karp related to the Rabbi the news that he was to be operated on and discussed with the Rabbi the chances of his surviving such surgery as well as the backup procedures and the fact that he would be the first human recipient of the mechanical heart substitute if the wedge procedure failed. There was no testimony given at the trial to refute Rabbi Wilkin's statements as to his conversations with Mr. Karp.

***

"Doctor Cooley testified that neither good medical standards nor his own personal practice would permit him to tell a patient that his condition was without hope and that he was going to die....

***

"Mr. Henry C. Reinhard, a St. Luke's Hospital administrator, testified that, on Thursday, April 3, 1969, he went to Mr. Karp's room where he found Mr. Karp alone and asked him if he had any questions regarding the surgical consent. They chatted for awhile and then Mr. Reinhard left the room. Mr. Reinhard further testified that on the day of surgery, Friday, April 4, 1969, he went to Mr. Karp's room where he found both Mr. Karp and Mrs. Karp present. He asked Mr. Karp if the signature on the following consent form as principal was his true signature wherein Mr. Karp replied affirmatively. Mr. Reinhard then asked Mrs. Karp if the signature as witness on the following consent form was her true signature wherein she replied affirmatively. Having explained to them that he wanted to verify the signature so that he could place his own name on the form, Mr. Reinhard witnessed, as Mrs. Karp had previously done, the following consent form:

> I, Haskell Karp, request and authorize Doctor Denton A. Cooley and such other surgeons as he may designate to perform upon me, in St.

Luke's Episcopal Hospital of Houston, Texas, cardiac surgery for advanced cardiac decompensation and myocardial insufficiency as a result of numerous coronary occlusions. The risk of this surgery has been explained to me. In the event cardiac function cannot be restored by excision of destroyed heart muscle and plastic reconstruction of the ventricle and death seems imminent, I authorize Doctor Cooley and his staff to remove my diseased heart and insert a mechanical cardiac substitute. I understand that this mechanical device will not be permanent and ultimately will require replacement by a heart transplant. I realize that this device has been tested in the Laboratory but has not been used to sustain a human being and that no assurance of success can be made. I expect the surgeons to exercise every effort to preserve my life through any of these means. No assurance has been made by anyone as to the results that may be obtained....

* * *

"In the early afternoon of April 4, 1969, Mr. Karp was rolled in the hall of the surgical ward. Doctor Arthur S. Keats, the anesthesiologist, passed the patient on his way to the operating room at approximately 1:55 p.m. Doctor Keats testified that he was alarmed by Mr. Karp's groaning and complaints of shortness of breath. Doctor Keats further testified that after observing Mr. Karp's coloring and profuse sweating it was his medical opinion that Mr. Karp would expire in the hallway if something was not done immediately. Doctor Keats sent word to Doctor Cooley that the operation should begin as soon as possible....

"Doctor Cooley then performed the wedge procedure in Mr. Karp's left ventricle. This surgery revealed that Mr. Karp's heart had extensive scarring and damage. Approximately 35 percent of the left ventricle was removed. After the surgery had been completed in its normal and customary fashion, the heart began to fibrillate. This was corrected by electrically shocking the heart. However, according to the only medical testimony given on the subject, the strength of the heart's contractions were not sufficient to sustain life in Mr. Karp. Therefore, according to backup procedures outlined in the written consent form, Doctor Cooley, assisted by Doctor Liotta, removed the heart and implanted the mechanical heart substitute.

"Mr. Karp regained consciousness and lived on the mechanical heart substitute for approximately 64 hours. During this period of time, Doctor Cooley and Mrs. Karp made public appeals through the news media for a human heart donor. On April 7, 1969, at 6:30

a.m., Mr. Karp underwent surgery to remove the mechanical heart
and to replace it with a human heart. His urine output was low after
the first surgery, and after the second, he became anuric despite all
measures to reverse the condition. Mr. Karp died on April 8, 1969,
at 3:15 p.m.

* * *

"After Mr. Karp's death, Mrs. Karp returned to her home in Illinois where she wrote numerous laudatory letters about Doctor
Cooley and also wrote an outline for a book about her husband's
medical experiences. This manuscript told of Mr. Karp's rapidly de-
teriorating physical condition before surgery and of both Mr. and
Mrs. Karp eagerness for Doctor Cooley to perform surgery on Mr.
Karp. Then in the fall of 1969, Mrs. Karp, individually and as Ex-
ecutor of the Estate of Haskell Karp, and their three sons filed suit
against Doctors Cooley and Liotta for damages sustained by Mr.
Karp and by plaintiffs under the Texas Wrongful Death Statute.
Plaintiffs alleged, among other things, that the consent to the operation was fraudulently obtained; that it was not an 'informed consent'; that under the circumstances the defendants were negligent in
performing the corrective surgery, implanting the mechanical heart,
and submitting the patient to the surgery for inserting the human
donor heart; and that by fraudulent deceptive practices Mrs. Karp
was used by defendants to secure a human heart donor.

* * *

"...[E]ach doctor must use his medical judgment as to whether
certain disclosures of risks would have an adverse effect on the patient so as to jeopardize the success of the proposed therapy. Doctor
Beasley, Doctor Hamaker, Doctor Keats, and Doctor Cooley all testified that it often is advisable to deliberately withhold information
from a patient that would unduly distress him. Doctor H.L Beasley
testified that this notation on Mr. Karp's chart of March 7, 1969, 'I
am not completely sold that this is a candidate for surgery...' had reference to Mr. Karp's poor emotional attitude towards his hospitalization. All the medical testimony stated that emotional attitude and
depression would affect what they would relate to a patient.

* * *

"It must also be considered at this point that the specially prepared consent form did relate some of the detailed information that

plaintiffs complain of, i.e. , 'I realize that this device has been tested in the laboratory but has not been used to sustain a human being and that no assurance of success can be made.' Texas law would require that a jury be instructed that Mr. Karp is charged with reading the consent even if in fact he did not....

"Under Texas law the jury would also have to have been instructed that Mrs. Karp's consent to the surgery was not required. Indeed, Mrs. Karp could not legally grant consent to surgery to be performed on her husband and, therefore, any information given to her or withheld from her could not have affected the informed consent of her husband....

"Acordingly, as to any issue of informed consent, a verdict must be directed for Doctor Cooley...."

***

QUESTIONS

1. What dangers exist with the use of substituted judgment?
2. When should a party other than the patient be consulted for informed consent? What makes a child knowledgeable enough that his/her views should be considered? Should the views of a child or an incompetent ever be considered?
3. To what extent can psychological needs be used to justify physical intervention that produces no physical benefit for the patient (and may even produce physical harm)?
4. Should local medical standards determine whether information provided a patient is sufficient for informed consent?
5. Can a conscious, normal adult in Mr. Karp's condition give informed consent? Can anyone who is hospitalized and facing the trauma of serious illness give informed consent?
6. If the risk of death resulting from a medical procedure is 20 percent, should a patient be told? 5 percent? 0.0001 percent?
7. Suppose a patient signs a blanket consent form which says, in effect, "I authorize the surgeon to do whatever he/she deems necessary." Should a court accept such a form as evidence of informed consent?
8. Should courts always examine the consent of minors or incompetents? If not, who will?

CHAPTER 4

THE RIGHT TO REFUSE TREATMENT
FOR RELIGIOUS REASONS

INTRODUCTION

THE First Amendment recognizes a fundamental right to the free exercise of religion. At times, that right interferes with treatment for patients. Suppose, for example, a blood transfusion is necessary to save a life of a patient who is a Jehovah's Witness. Jehovah's Witnesses believe that God has forbidden Christians from having transfusions. Relying on Acts of the Apostles, and Leviticus, they must "abstain...from blood" and from "eating the blood."[1] To a devout Jehovah's Witness, such words mean that they must refrain from receiving blood transfusions. The patient, as a result, will refuse the life-saving transfusion.

This case differs from a typical right-to-die case. It is not a situation where death is being held away from a hopelessly dying patient, nor is this the type of right-to-die case where one who is severely defective is being allowed to die by withholding necessary medical treatment. This issue often involves a normal adult who is refusing medical treatment because of religious opposition to the treatment and not because of any desire to die.

When such cases present themselves, judges usually issue court orders that allow the medical procedure in spite of the opposition of the patient. However, the judge often has to be convinced that the treatment is necessary to save a life. It is unlikely that a judge would allow interference with First Amendment freedoms in the absence of a "compelling state interest." Nonessential treatments would lack the compelling quality that is present where life is at stake. Judge Skelly Wright explained his reasoning in a decision where he order a transfusion for a twenty-five-year-old mother who refused a transfusion for religious reasons. "To refuse to act, only to find later that the law

---

[1] *Jehovah's Witnesses in State of Washington v. King County Hospital,* 278 F. Supp. at 502 (1967).

required action, was a risk I was unwilling to accept. I determined to act on the side of life."[2]

These decisions can be extremely difficult ones to make. Judge Jacob Markowitz was obviously torn when he ordered a transfusion for a mother of six: "Never before has my judicial robe weighed so heavily on my shoulders."[3] Markowitz recognized that on one scale of the balance was the life of the patient. However, on the other scale were very important interests as well, such as the interest of the patient in religious liberty, the patient's right of privacy, and the patient's right to control his/her body against invasive medical treatments.

Courts usually justify their decisions by arguing that while there may be an absolute right of religious belief, religious exercise is subject to limitations. Similarly, privacy and bodily control rights are not absolute. Weighed against these limited rights, the state's interest in maintaining life is dominant. However, an incompetent person may be forced to exercise his/her right to die. If so, can a competent person be forced to live?

Another problem raised in this chapter involves parental refusal of medical treatment for children due to religious beliefs. It is frequently argued that guardians have no right to impose religious judgments that would lead to the deaths of minors and incompetents.[4] Yet, some courts have held that guardians may make non-religious judgments that lead to the deaths of minors and incompetents.[5] In cases involving religion, the judge will usually allow the state to act in the place of parents and will order the necessary medical procedure. The courts have generally held that religious justifications cannot be legitimately used to endanger the welfare of a child.

This nation is one which has prided itself on its diverse people. That diversity in its population means that the United States has a great variety of religious views. The result is that the conflicts between medicine and religious groups are likely to remain. However,

---

[2]Rothenberg, Leslie S.: Demands for life and requests for death: The judicial dilemma. In McMullin, Ernan (Ed.): *Death and Decision* (Boulder, Westview, 1978, p. 135).

[3]Rothenberg, op cit., p. 137.

[4]*Jehovah's Witnesses in State of Washington v. King County Hospital,* 278 F. Supp. 488 (1967).

[5]For example, the unreported Indiana Supreme Court case, *In Re Baby Doe* which is discussed in Chapter 7, "The Right To Die."

advances in medical technology can change the specific issues around which conflicts occur. In the days prior to widespread blood transfusions, the conflicts between Jehovah's Witnesses and physicians were rare. One died if one desperately needed a transfusion. As blood transfusions became routine, however, conflicts between Jehovah's Witnesses and the medical community naturally increased.

This medical-legal problem may become moot as synthetic blood becomes available. Researchers have been experimenting with three categories of synthetic blood replacements: (1) stroma-free hemoglobin, (2) oxygen-binding chelates, and (3) perfluorochemicals.[6] Of these, perfluorochemicals currently have the most potential and have been used in clinical trials in Japan and in the United States.[7] The fluorocarbon substance can carry large amounts of oxygen, and it is widely believed that widespread use of synthetic blood is likely within the next few years.

---

[6]Leser, Doborah Rimmer:Synthetic blood:A future alternative (*American Journal of Nursing, 82*:452-455, 1982).
[7]Gonzalez, Elizabeth Rasche:Fluosol a special boon to Jehovah's Witnesses (*The Journal of the American Medical Association, 243*:720, 724, 1980).

APPLICATION OF PRESIDENT
AND DIRECTORS OF GEORGETOWN COLLEGE

(U.S. Court of Appeals, 1964)
331 F. 2d 1000

May a woman be forced to undergo blood transfusions against the religious beliefs of both herself and her spouse?

J. SKELLY WRIGHT, CIRCUIT JUDGE:

* * *

"Mrs. Jones was brought to the hospital by her husband for emergency care, having lost two-thirds of her body's blood supply from a ruptured ulcer. She had no personal physician and relied solely on the hospital staff. She was a total hospital responsibility. It appeared that the patient, aged twenty-five, mother of a seven-month-old child, and her husband were both Jehovah's Witnesses, the teachings of which sect, according to their interpretation, prohibited the injection of blood into the body. When death without blood became imminent, the hospital sought the adivce of counsel, who applied to the District Court in the name of the hospital for permission to administer blood. Judge Tamm of the District Court denied the application and counsel immediately applied to me, as a member of the Court of Appeals, for an appropriate writ.

"I called the hospital by telephone and spoke with Doctor Westura, Chief Medical Resident, who confirmed the representations made by counsel. I thereupon proceeded with counsel to the hospital, where I spoke to Mr. Jones, the husband of the patient. He advised me that, on religious grounds, he would not approve a blood transfusion for his wife. He said, however, that if the court ordered the transfusion, the responsibility was not his. I advised Mr. Jones to obtain counsel immediately. He thereupon went to the telephone and returned in 10 or 15 minutes to advise that he had taken the matter up with his church and that he had decided that he did not want counsel.

"I asked permission of Mr. Jones to see his wife. This he readily granted. Prior to going to the patient's room, I again conferred with Doctor Westura and several other doctors assigned to the case. All confirmed that the patient would die without blood and that there was a better than 50 percent chance of saving her life with it. Unanimously, they strongly recommended it. I then went inside the patient's room. Her appearance confirmed the urgency which had been represented to me. I tried to communicate with her, advising her again as to what the doctors had said. The only audible reply I could hear was 'Against my will.' It was obvious that the woman was not in a mental condition to make a decision. I was reluctant to press her because of the seriousness of her condition and because I felt that to suggest repeatedly the imminence of death without blood might place a strain on her religious convictions. I asked her whether she would oppose the blood transfusion if the Court allowed it. She indicated, as best I could make out, that it would then not be her responsibility.

"I returned to the doctor's room where some ten to twelve doctors were congregated, along with the husband and counsel for the hospital. The President of Georgetown University, Father Bunn, appeared and pleaded with Mr. Jones to authorize the hospital to save his wife's life with a blood transfusion. Mr. Jones replied that the Scriptures say that we should not drink blood, and consequently his religion prohibited transfusions. The doctors explained to Mr. Jones that a blood transfusion is totally different from drinking blood in that the blood physically goes into a different part and through a different process in the body. Mr. Jones was unmoved. I thereupon signed the order allowing the hospital to administer such transfusions as the doctors should determine were necessary to save her life.

***

"...Mrs. Jones was *in extremis* and hardly *compos mentis* at the time in question; she was as little able competently to decide for herself as any child would be. Under the circumstances it may well be the duty of a court of general jurisdiction, such as the United States District Court for the District of Columbia, to assume the responsibility of guardianship for her, as for a child, at least to the extent of authorizing treatment to save her life. And if ... a parent has no power to forbid the saving of his child's life, *a fortiori,* the husband of the patient here had no right to order the doctors to treat his wife in a way so that she would die.

"...The state, as *parens patriae,* will not allow a parent to abandon a child, and so it should not allow this most ultimate of voluntary abandonments. The patient had a responsibility to the community to care for her infant. Thus the people had an interest in preserving the life of the mother.

***

"If self-homicide is a crime, there is no exception to the law's command for those who believe the crime to be divinely ordained.... But whether attempted suicide is a crime is in doubt in some jurisdictions, including the District of Columbia.

"The Gordian knot of this suicide question may be cut by the simple fact that Mrs. Jones did not want to die. Her voluntary presence in the hospital as a patient seeking medical help testified to this. Death, to Mrs. Jones, was not a religously commanded goal, but an unwanted side effect of a religious scruple. There is no question here of interfering with one whose religious convictions counsel his death, like the Buddhist monks who set themselves afire. Nor are we faced with the question of whether the state should intervene to reweigh the relative values of life and death, after the individual has weighed them for himself and found life wanting. Mrs. Jones wanted to live.

"A third set of considerations involved the position of the doctors and the hospital. Mrs. Jones was their responsibility to treat. The hospital doctors had the choice of administering the proper treatment or letting Mrs. Jones die in the hospital bed, thus exposing themselves and the hospital to the risk of civil and criminal liability in either case.... It is not clear just where a patient would derive her authority to command her doctor to treat her under limitations which would produce death. The patient's counsel suggests that this authority is part of constitutionality protected liberty. But neither the principle that life and liberty are inalienable rights, nor the principle of liberty of religion, provides an easy answer to the question whether the state can prevent martyrdom. Moreover, Mrs. Jones had no wish to be a martyr....

"The final, and compelling, reason for granting the emergency writ was that a life hung in the balance. There was no time for research and reflection. Death could have mooted the cause in a matter of minutes if action were not taken to preserve the status quo. To refuse to act, only to find later that the law required action, was a risk I was unwilling to accept. I determined to act on the side of life."

APPLICATION OF PRESIDENT
AND DIRECTORS OF GEORGETOWN COLLEGE (REHEARING)

(U.S. Court of Appeals, 1964)
331 F. 2d 1010

A rehearing of Judge Wright's order was requested before the entire D.C. Circuit Court of Appeals.

PER CURIAM:

"Upon consideration of a pleading styled 'Petition for Rehearing En Banc' in the above-entitled matter and an opposition thereto, it is ordered by the court en banc that said petition is denied."

(Judge Washington concurred. Judge Danaher would dismiss for lack of a case and controversy.)

JUDGE MILLER DISSENTING:

* * *

"It seems clear to me, however, that the matter did not properly come before this court and that, had it been duly presented on appeal, one judge of this court was not authorized to make a summary disposition of the matter on the merits... no action was filed in the District Court...no appeal was filed in this court; and...had there been an actual appeal, a single appellate judge was not authorized to act.

* * *

"I do not mean to impugn the motives of our colleague who signed these orders. He was impelled, I am sure, by humanitarian impulses and doubtless was himself under considerable strain because of the critical situation in which he had become involved. In the interval of about an hour and twenty minutes between the appearance of the attorneys at his chambers and the signing of the order at the hospital, the judge had no opportunity for research as to the substantive legal problems and procedural questions involved. He should not have been asked to act in these circumstances.

"I suggest it is not correct to suppose that, where there is a serious emergency in life, a judge of a district or a circuit court may act to set it, regardless of whether he is empowered by law to do so. This situation shows the truth of the adage that hard cases make bad law."

(Judge Bastian and Burger joined in the dissent.)

JUDGE BURGER DISSENTING:

* * *

"...The choice between violating the patient's convictions of conscience and accepting her decision was hardly an easy one.

However, since it is not disputed that the patient and her husband volunteered to sign a waiver to relieve the hospital of any liability for the consequences of failure to effect the transfusion, any claim to a protected right in the economic damage sphere would appear unsupported.

"Can a legally protected right arise out of some other duty-right of the hospital toward a patient, such as a moral obligation to preserve life at all costs?

"For me it is difficult to construct an actionable or legally protected right out of this relationship. The affirmative enforcement of a right growing out of a possible moral duty of the hospital toward a patient does not seem to meet the standards of justiciability especially when the only remedy is judicial compulsion touching the sensitive area of conscience and religious belief."

* * *

UNITED STATES V. GEORGE

(U.S. District Court, 1965)
239 F. Supp. 752

Elishas George, a thirty-nine-year-old father of four children, voluntarily admitted himself to a hospital for treatment of a bleeding ulcer. Serious bleeding suggested a need for blood transfusions, which George refused for religious reasons. Both he and his wife signed releases which relieved the hospital and its employees for any injury which might result from lack of transfusions. Nevertheless, a court order was sought which would grant permission to the hospital to administer transfusions to George.

ZAMPANO, DISTRICT JUDGE:

* * *

"The medical testimony was clear the blood loss was so great that standard medical care dictated that administration immediately of at least five pints of whole blood. The laboratory tests indicated he had already lost 60% to 65% of his red blood cells. His condition was grave, and any further bleeding, without blood transfusion, would most likely lead to shock and probable death. Psychiatric reports indicated the patient showed a lack of concern for life, and a somewhat fatalistic attitude about his condition was described as 'a variant of suicide.'

"Mr. George appeared to the Court to be coherent, rational and rather strong. However, doctors in attendance agreed his outward appearance was deceiving and his internal condition was most serious. When the Court introduced himself, George's first remarks were that he would not agree to be transfused but would in no way resist a court order permitting it, because it would be the Court's will and not his own. His 'conscience was clear,' and the responsibility for the act was 'upon the Court's conscience.' He stated he would rather die than agree to a transfusion. The Court advised George it had no power to force a transfusion upon him, and he was free to resist the transfusion, even by the rather simple physical maneuver of placing his hand over the area to be injected by the needle. George stated he would 'in no way' resist the doctor's actions once the Court's order was signed.

"Mrs. George, citing certain passages from the Bible, was adamant in her opposition to the transfusions. She insisted that the Court had no right to order the transfusion in violation of their religious beliefs. Two other Jehovah's Witnesses, visiting the patient, concurred in Mrs. George's remarks.

"The patient's mother, Mrs. George, not a member of the sect, informed the Court her son has been a Jehovah's Witness for two years, and she favored the transfusions.

"The Court thereupon signed the order allowing the hospital to 'administer such blood transfusions as are in the opinion of the physicians in attendance necessary to save the patient's life.' Moreover, the Court ordered another hearing on the motion on March 26, 1965, or 'at such time as may be requested by the patient, his wife, or their legal representative.' To date, neither the Georges nor their legal representative have petitioned the Court to dissolve the order.

***

"...In the difficult realm of religious liberty it is often assumed only the religious conscience is imperiled. Here, however, the doctor's conscience and professional oath must also be respected. In the present case, the patient voluntarily submitted himself to and insisted upon medical care. Simultaneously he sought to dictate to treating physicians a course of treatment amounting to medical malpractice. To require these doctors to ignore the mandates of their own conscience, even in the name of free religious exercise, cannot be justified under these circumstances. The patient may knowingly decline treatment, but he may not demand mistreatment. Therefore, this Court, as Judge Wright, 'determined to act on the side of life' in the pending emergency....

"The Court was informed that a series of transfusions have commenced since the signing of the order. No request has been made by the Georges or their counsel to test the legality of the order. However, on March 22, 1965, the government filed the present motion to dissolve the temporary restraining order and to withdraw the complaint. Supported by affidavits, the government alleges that the patient is no longer *in extremis* and is now sufficiently physicially rehabilitated to determine with reflection and study the propriety of continued blood transfusions for his own complete recovery.

"Accordingly, the motion is granted."

JOHN F. KENNEDY MEMORIAL HOSPITAL V. HESTON

(New Jersey Supreme Court, 1971)
279 A. 2d 670

Unconscious from an automobile accident, Delores Heston, a twenty-two-year-old, single female, required blood transfusions if her life was to be saved. Delores's mother refused permission to transfuse blood based on religious beliefs. May the courts require transfusion?

CHIEF JUSTICE WEINTRAUB DELIVERED THE OPINION OF THE COURT:

***

"It seems correct to say there is not a constitutional right to choose to die....

"Nor is constitutional right established by adding that one's religious faith ordains his death. Religious beliefs are absolute, but conduct in pursuance of religious beliefs is not wholly immune from governmental restraint...."

* * *

"...The question is whether the State may authorize force to prevent death or may tolerate the use of force by others to that end. Indeed, the issue is not solely between the State and Miss Heston, for the controversy is also between Miss Heston and a hospital and staff who did not seek her out and upon whom the dictates of her faith will fall as a burden. Hospitals exist to aid the sick and the injured. The medical and nursing professions are consecrated to preserving life. That is their professional creed. To them, a failure to use a simple, established procedure in the circumstances of this case would be malpractice, however, the law may characterize that failure because of the patient's private convictions. A surgeon should not be asked to operate under the strain of knowing that a transfusion may not be administered even though medically required to save his patient. The hospital and its staff should not be required to decide whether the patient is or continues to be competent to make a judgment upon the subject, or whether the release tendered by the patient or a member of his family will protect them from civil responsibility. The hospital could hardly avoid the problem by compelling the removal of a dying patient, and Miss Heston's family made no effort to take her elsewhere.

"When the hospital and staff are thus involuntary hosts and their interests are pitted against the belief of the patient, we think it reasonable to resolve the problem by permitting the hospital and its staff to pursue their functions according to their professional standards. The solution sides with life, the conservation of which is, we think, a matter of State interest. A prior application to a court is appropriate if time permits it, although in the nature of the emergency the only question that can be explored satisfactorily is whether death will probably ensue if medical procedures are not followed. If a court finds, as the trial court did, that death will likely follow unless a transfusion is administered, the hospital and the physician should be permitted to follow that medical procedure."

* * *

MITCHELL V. DAVIS

(Texas Court of Civil Appeals, 1947)
205 S. W. 2d 812

A child was removed from the home because it received inadequate medical care. Rather than traditional care, the mother cared for the child primarily with home remedies and by praying.

YOUNG, JUSTICE:

* * *

"...There was evidence that Leroy was a normally alert and energetic boy before August, 1946, when he grew ill, progressively becoming worse; right knee swelling, face pale, moving about with difficulty and using crutches. During the first six weeks of fall term, he attended school about one-half of the time; second six weeks, about one-sixth of the time, and last six weeks, not at all. Prior to suit, he was observed to move about with much pain; appearance in courtroom contrasting greatly with that previous to illness, according to Mrs. Albrech, school nurse. She stated that he had lost considerable weight, was thinner, paler, eyes red-rimmed, knee greatly swollen, as was ankle; not appearing alert, energetic or interested. Such was the report of this witness from several visits up to December, 1946. Doctor Bumpass, family physician, was called to the Mitchell home on February 3 (after filing of suit), testifying that Leroy was probably suffering from arthritis or complications following rheumatic fever; no positive diagnosis being obtainable without complete clinical tests and medical observation; the mother being then advised to secure the services of an orthopedist. Mrs. Mitchell refused to further consult a regular physician, though frequently urged to do so, continuing to rely on home remedies and prayer. During the trial she refused to permit a commitment of the boy to a hospital where he could receive diagnosis and treatment by the family physician free of charge. Prior to trial, the mother took appellant to a chiropractor and an osteopath, who were unable to positively diagnose his condition (except that X-rays indicated a calcium deficiency), and who failed to recommend or suggest a cure or course of treatment. In this connection, an excerpt from the testimony of Mrs. Albrech, school nurse, who called at the home on November 26, 1946, is somewhat revealing: 'Q. Did you have any futher conversation with Mrs. Mitchell at that time with reference to medical treatment? A. Yes, sir. I asked her if she had consulted a doctor on this particular case and she said she hadn't and furthermore she didn't think it was necessary so long as she was praying for him, that this condition had persisted since school opened. She told me it started last summer before school started and at times it was far worse and I should have seen him sometimes when he was in far worse condition than that; that sometimes he couldn't get out of bed and they prayed and when she and the child prayed he had strength to get up and go and sometimes he would be out playing and come in crying, in the mother's words, "with tears streaming down his face," and asking her to pray and do something for him and at one time she was sewing at the sewing machine and he sank to the floor and begged her to do something and she got down on her knees by the side of the child and prayed.'

"Mrs. Mitchell, mother, on the other hand stoutly denied any charge of child neglect, it being evident that her rejection of orthodox medical treatment and adherence to home remedies and prayer, was because of religious belief in the fact of Divine Healing and her absolute faith in the power of religion to overcome all physical ailments and disease.

"The legal point of interference with the freedom of religious worship is thus raised. Says the United States Supreme Court, in *Reynolds v. United States*...: 'Laws are made for the government of actions, and while they cannot interfere with mere religious beliefs and opinions, they may with practice....'

"The case narrows, therefore, to the fact question of neglect.... We have given due consideration to the argument made of the mother's natural and constitutional right to appellant's care and custody. While a considerable amount of discretion is vested in a parent charged with the duty of maintaining and bringing up her children, the right of appellant and his mother here to live their own lives in their own way is not absolute. 'While ordinarily the natural parents are entitled to the custody and care of their child, this is not an absolute unconditional right. The State has such an interest in the welfare of its citizens as will authorize the enactment of suitable legislation by which the State may assume the custody of children and the parents may be deprived of the custody thereof where the parents abandon the children or neglect them in such manner as to cause them to become a public charge, or where the parents otherwise prove to be unsuitable....

"Onerous as this order of custody may appear to the parties herein complaining, its entry was solely in the interest of appellant.

It is not irrevocable, yielding always to changed conditions. The medical treatment outlined and recommended by the mother's own physician, followed by a reasonable cooperation on her part with juvenile authorities in the matter of appellant's physical welfare, will doubtless conclude this unhappy incident and result in his restoration to the usual routine of family life. But as the record now stands, the order of custody must be affirmed."

JEFFERSON V. GRIFFIN SPALDING COUNTY HOSPITAL

(Supreme Court of Georgia, 1981)
274 S.E. 2d 457

Mrs. Jesse Jefferson was pregnant and had a complete placenta previa. That is, the afterbirth was between the baby and the birth canal. Her examining physician recommended a caesarean section prior to the onset of labor. Mrs. Jefferson refused the surgery and any blood transfusions on the basis of her religious beliefs. The state alleged child deprivation and sought temporary custody of the unborn child. The Butts County Juvenile Court, acting as both a superior court or equity court and a juvenile court, granted custody on the following grounds.

PER CURIAM:

* * *

"Based on the evidence presented, the Court finds that Jessie Mae Jefferson is due to begin labor at any moment. There is a 99 to 100 percent certainty that the unborn child will die if she attempts to have the child by vaginal delivery. There is a 99 to 100 percent chance that the child will live if the baby is delivered by Caesarean section prior to the beginning of the labor. There is a 50 percent chance that Mrs. Jefferson herself will die if vaginal delivery is attempted. There is an almost 100 percent chance that Mrs. Jefferson will survive if a delivery by Caesarean section is done prior to the beginning of labor.

"Mrs. Jefferson and her husband have refused and continue to refuse to give consent to a Caesarean section. This refusal is based entirely on the religious beliefs of Mr. and Mrs. Jefferson. They are of the view that the Lord has healed her body and that whatever happens to the child will be the Lord's will.

"Based on these findings, the Court concludes and finds as a matter of law that this child is a viable human being and entitled to the protection of the Juvenile Court Code of Georgia. The Court concludes that this child is without the proper parental care and subsistence necessary to his or her physical life and health.

"Temporary custody of the unborn child is hereby granted to the State of Georgia Department of Human Resources and the Butts County Department of Family and Children Services. The department shall have full authority to make all decisions, including giving consent to the surgical delivery appertaining to the birth of this child. The temporary custody of the Department shall terminate when the child has been successfully brought from its mother's body into the world or until the child dies, whichever shall happen."

***

(The state supreme court denied a motion to stay the Juvenile Court's order. All the justices concurred in the denial.)

JUSTICE HILL CONCURS, JOINED BY JUSTICE MARSHALL:

"The power of a court to order a competent adult to submit to surgery is exceedingly limited. Indeed, until this unique case arose, I would have thought such power to be nonexistent...."

***

"In denying the stay of the trial court's order and thereby clearing the way for immediate reexamination by sonogram and probability for surgery, we weighed the right of the mother to practice her religion and to refuse surgery on herself, against her unborn child's right to live. We found in favor of her child's right to live."

***

JUSTICE SMITH CONCURS:

"The free exercise of religion is, of course, one of our most precious freedoms. The courts have, however, drawn a distinction between the free exercise of religious belief which is constitutionally protected against any infringement and religious practices that are inimical or detrimental to public health or welfare which are not...."

***

"In the instant case, it appears that there is no less burdensome alternative for preserving the life of a fully developed fetus than requiring its mother to undergo surgery against her religious convictions.... However, the state's compelling interest in preserving the life of this fetus is beyond dispute.... Moreover, the medical evidence indicates that the risk to the fetus and the mother presented by a Caesarean section would be minimal, whereas, in the absence of surgery, the fetus would almost certainly die and the mother's chances of survival would be no better than 50 percent....

"We deal here with an apparent life and death emergency: questions relating to the jurisdiction of the lower court are not our primary concern....

"I believe the legislature intended that the juvenile courts exercise jurisdiction only where a child has seen the light of day. I am aware of no child deprivation proceeding wherein the child was unborn....

"...The trial court, in an attempt to cover all possible ground, rendered its judgment, 'both as a Juvenile Court and under the broad powers of the Superior Court of Butts County.' As the trial court's action was a proper exercise of its equitable jurisdiction with respect to both the mother and the fetus... and its decision on the merits a correct one, I fully concur in the denial of appellant's motion for stay..."

QUESTIONS

1. If people have a right to die, why not for religious reasons? Or, does the right to die only exist in cases of persons who suffer terminal illnesses? If so, why was Baby Doe allowed to die (see the introductory comments for Chap. 7).

2. If one should err in favor of life as Judge Wright did in *Application of the President and Directors of Georgetown Hospital,* should such a decision be reached in all questions where one may choose between life and death? If one does always err in favor of life, does that mean that the doctrine of wrongful life is an invalid one (see Chap. 8)?

3. If parents have the right to make major life-and-death decisions for their children (e.g. the *Baby Doe* case and, in a different sense, *In Re Philip B.*), why can't they make it on religious grounds?

4. *Mitchell v. Davis* shows hostility to nontraditional medical treatments. Would it have been neglect if a traditional physician, rather than God, was regularly consulted for care of the child?

5. Would the Court's decision have been different in *Jefferson v. Griffen Spalding County Hospital* if the fetus had been defective? If the fetus had been born defective, would the court have been guilty of causing a wrongful life?

6. In such conflicts between religion and the state, is there a kind of implied conspiracy which may sometimes be at work? That is, if a person wants to insure that no offensive medical treatment is forced upon him/her, why go to a hospital? Of course, in some cases, the patient may not realize that such offensive treatments will be thought necessary. However, a patient who knows he/she is bleeding to death might well realize that a hospital will try to perform blood transfusions. By entering a hospital in such cases, is the patient implicitly saying, "I don't want to die, force me to live by ignoring my religious convictions"? Might some of the judges in the readings assume the patient makes such a plea?

7. Why would spouses and relatives be consulted for their views on a religiously offensive treatment? Especially in cases where the patient is responsive, isn't his/her objection to the treatment the only view that should be considered by the court?

8. Could the court overrule religious objections in non-life-threatening situations where it was felt better health would be promoted by performing a particular medical procedure? Would "better health" be a compelling interest to be promoted by the state? The line between life-threatening and non-life-threatening situations may not always be clear. For example, a smallpox vaccination may not have clearly been required for life — though for a long time it was essential in preventing major outbreaks of the disease. Could not a person have been compelled to be vaccinated against their religious beliefs?

CHAPTER 5

THE PATIENT IN CONFINEMENT

INTRODUCTION

IN recent years, courts have become very concerned with the treatment of confined persons. Prisoners, for example, until recently were often held to be civilly dead. Civil death meant that they lost most rights, including the right to complain to the courts about the conditions of their confinement. The new concern for prisoners' rights, however, has opened up vast areas for prisoner litigation. One of those areas deals with the medical treatment of prisoners. Among the primary medical treatment concerns are the issues of what can be done to a prisoner against his/her will and what rights to medical treatment the prisoner may assert. Similar issues are also of judicial concern in reference to the rights of those confined to mental institutions.

Often, the judicial assertion of rights for the institutionalized is accompanied by great controversy. There are several reasons for the controversy; one involves cost considerations. Recognition of a prisoner's right to medical treatment can be extremely expensive, an expense that must be borne by the taxpayers. Prisoners are far from a popular or politically influential group. The fact that citizens have to pay higher taxes or do without other services in order to maintain those who have chosen to burden society usually does not strike a responsive chord among the electorate or among politicians. Recognition of prisoners' rights to refuse treatment may also upset the routine of prison life. Thus, not only might great expense be involved, but a recognition of such rights may cause administrative burdens.

It should also be noted that in many cases the interests of prisoners have so long been ignored that to recognize a right to refuse treatment or a right to adequate medical treatment is to require a completely new way of thinking about prisons and prisoners. For those accustomed to the old-fashioned approach of "lock them up and ignore them," cases which stress the rights of prisoners must be especially upsetting.

While those confined to mental institutions are not as politically unpopular as those in prison, a recognition of the rights of the mentally ill also raises cost concerns. The rights of the mentally ill are faced with another competing concern as well. Is it proper to recognize that mentally ill persons have personal autonomy? Can they be given a right to make choices about their medical treatment? It can be argued that they are not competent to make choices about their treatment. Thus, to give them choices is to make their treatment and recovery more difficult and is therefore a bad medical practice. Nevertheless, courts are providing some recognition of the personal autonomy rights of those confined to mental institutions.

UNITED STATES V. CROWDER

(United States Court of Appeals, District of Columbia, 1976)
543 F. 2d 312

May surgery be performed on a prisoner to recover evidence?

CIRCUIT JUDGE ROBB:

* * *

"On the afternoon of December 18, 1970, Doctor James E. Bowman, a dentist, was murdered in his office. Death was caused by a gunshot wound entering his chest and coursing through his heart. A caliber .32 slug, which apparently had passed through his body, was found in his underwear. The police found a caliber .32 Smith & Wesson revolver on the ground, across the street from the doctor's office. The revolver contained four expended rounds and two live rounds. It had been kept in the doctor's office and was registered to his wife.

"On December 23, 1970, the police arrested one Sandra Toomer, charged her with the murder, and she in turn implicated Crowder. She told the police that she and Crowder had gone to the doctor's office intending to rob him. When Crowder confronted the doctor with a toy pistol, she said, a scuffle ensued, she ran, and she then heard gunshots. Rejoining her, Crowder told her he had been shot in his arm and his left leg, but he thought he had killed the doctor. She observed Crowder's wounds.

"Acting on the information given Sandra Toomer, the police arrested Crowder. They noted that his right wrist and left thigh were bandaged. They took him to D.C. General Hospital where x-rays disclosed a bullet lodged in his right forearm and another in his left thigh. The bullets appeared to be caliber .32 slugs. Crowder refused to be treated for his wounds.

"As might be expected, the police and the prosecutor thought it important to determine whether the slugs in Crowder's arm and leg had been fired from the Bowman revolver. Accordingly, on February 10, 1971, the United States Attorney presented to Chief Judge Curran of the District Court an application for an order authorizing the surgical removal of the bullet from Crowder's arm. The application was supported by an affidavit from Detective Richardson of the Homicide Unit...narrating in substance the evidence that we have set out. In addition, the United States Attorney tendered an affidavit from Doctor Marcus Goumas, Senior Medical Officer at the District of Columbia jail where Crowder was incarcerated. Doctor Goumas affirmed that x-rays of Crowder's left thigh and right forearm revealed the presence of metallic foreign bodies resembling bullets. Doctor Goumas expressed the opinion 'that it would be medically inadvisable to remove surgically the slug from Mr. Crowder's left thigh because such a procedure might cause the reduction of use or function of his left leg.' The slug in his right forearm, however, is lying superficially under the skin. It is therefore my medical opinion, based upon reasonable medical certainty, that the surgical removal of the slug would not involve any harm or risk of injury to Mr. Crowder's arm or hand or the use thereof. The surgical removal of the slug would be considered as minor surgery. If authorized, it will be performed in accordance with accepted medical practices by one or more surgeons in an operating room at D.C. General Hospital under a local anesthetic. Mr. Crowder will probably be hospitalized for a few days in D.C. General Hospital after this surgery to guard against possible infection.

"The United States Attorney's application came on for hearing before Chief Judge Curran on February 10. The defendant Crowder appeared with counsel and objected to the entry of the requested order....

"Chief Judge Curran found probable cause to believe that Crowder murdered Doctor Bowman and that 'evidence of instrumentality of that offense' was located in Crowder's right forearm and left thigh.

"On the basis of his findings...the judge ordered:

1. That the Superintendent of the District of Columbia General Hospital, or his authorized representative or representatives, shall remove from the right forearm of James L. Crowder the foreign matter disclosed by x-rays and positively believed to be a .32 slug;

2. That such removal is to be done at the District of Columbia General Hospital with accepted medical procedures, with due regard given to the health and preservation of life of James L. Crowder;

3. That if at any time during the course of the removal procedures danger to the life of James L. Crowder develops, such removal procedures shall cease and such other steps as may be necessary shall be taken to protect the health and life of James L. Crowder; and

4. That after removal of the foreign matter, such matter shall be turned over to an authorized representative of the Metropolitan Police Department, who is to make a return to the Court in accordance with the requirements of Rule 41 of the Federal Rules of Criminal Procedure.

5. The defendant shall not tamper with or disturb the wound in his right forearm, or remove, destroy or dispose of the bullet lodged therein.

"A petition for a writ of prohibition against the execution of Chief Judge Curran's order was denied by this court on March 2, 1971.... On April 9, 1971, at D.C. General Hospital, Doctor Henry H. Balch removed the bullet from Crowder's right arm. Thereafter, a motion to suppress the bullet as evidence was filed by Crowder....

* * *

"The district judge overruled the motion to suppress the bullet.

"As the Supreme Court observed in *Schmerber v. California*,...'the Fourth Amendment's proper function is to constrain, not against all intrusions as such, but against intrusions which are not justified in the circumstances, or which are made in an improper manner.' When this standard is applied to the facts we have outlined, we think the conclusion is irresistible that the removal of the bullet from Crowder's arm was reasonable and proper.

"In the first place, before acting to retrieve the bullet, the prosecuting authorities presented the matter to Chief Judge Curran, a neutral and detached magistrate, for his decision. An adversary hearing was held at which Crowder appeared with counsel. The appellant concedes that probable cause was established. Chief Judge Curran's order was carefully drawn and hedged so as to protect Crowder's health and life; thus the order directed that only the bullet in Crowder's forearm be removed, leaving untouched the bullet in his thigh, and that every medical and surgical precaution be taken.

"As the skilled and experienced surgeon who performed the operation testified 'maximum precautions' were taken when the bullet was removed, 'we bent over backwards.' The bullet, which was small, close to the skin and easily felt, was extracted by gentle squeezing after an incision an inch long had been made. Less than five cc.'s of blood were lost, an amount smaller than may be taken in a premarital examination. The entire operation took ten minutes. In the opinion of the surgeon, the risk was 'negligible' and in fact there were no complications. Although Crowder was kept in the 'care ward' for four or five days, the procedures did not require such treatment. Had Crowder been a private patient, he would have been discharged immediately and told he might go back to work; the care ward precaution was imposed only because the surgeon 'bent over backwards,' no doubt having in mind the possibility of future legal complications.

We do not find in these procedures, as the Supreme Court did in *Rochin v. California*...and the defendant does here, any conduct 'so brutal and so offensive to human dignity' that it 'shocks the conscience....' We think those procedures were reasonable and justified in the circumstances....

If the defendant's argument is sound, then no intrusion into a man's body that goes beyond a needle prick can ever be authorized by a court. We cannot agree that this is or ought to be the law. In our opinion the prosecuting authorities in this case made an intelligent and commendable effort to comply with the law; they resorted to 'skillful and imaginative legal planning, bottomed upon cooperative utilization, rather than utter disregard, of judicial power, and designed to achieve legitimate ends....' "

***

Circuit Judge Robinson, Joined by Chief Judge Bazelon and Circuit Judge Wright, Dissenting:

"In my view, the District Court erred...in admitting into evidence the bullet which had been surgically extracted from Crowder's forearm....

***

"...Use of a scalpel to make a cut an inch long and a quarter-inch deep into the subcutaneous fat of the arm is not 'commonplace.' Unlike the blood tests and perhaps a few other very minor medical procedures which most Americans regularly and unhesitatingly undergo, surgical incisions entail preoperative anesthesia, postoperative pain killers, stitches and permanent scars. They involve much more in the way of physical and mental discomfort and anxiety. They pose significantly higher risks of infection and postsurgery complications, and an immensely greater personal affront.

"Moreover, in weighing individual privacy against public needs for evidence of crime, surgery balances the scales much more closely. The measurement of alcoholic levels with blood testing is perhaps the most reliable method of identifying — or exonerating — the unfortunately large number of people daily suspected of driving while intoxicated. It may itself be a worthwhile deterrent of more drunk driving than we have. By contrast, the comparative rarity of surgical explorations for evidence of crimes casts doubt on their need for purposes of detection or deterrence. Surely in the instant case the bullet retrieved from Crowder's arm was far less crucial in the endeavor to bring him to book than blood tests generally are in convicting drunk drivers. Here the evidentiary significance of the bullet lay solely in its tendency to show that Crowder was present at the scene of the crime — a fact never in dispute at Crowder's trial.

"Even more fundamentally, the constitutionally indispensible balancing of the societal interest in effective law enforcement and the individual interest in personal integrity assumes an entirely different dimension in surgery cases. One's body simply cannot be equated with his car, his clothing, or even his home as a repository of evidence. By the same token, a surgical entry cannot be treated as just another police search. To me it seems incontrovertible that, with its marked intensification of risk, pain, scarring and indignity, a surgical invasion of the body cannot be likened to the needle puncture....

"I am unable to view calmly this court's action in sanctioning new and far greater bodily exploration than the ubiquitous needle insertion permitted in *Schmerber*. By extending that decision to all instances of so-called 'minor surgery,' the court paves the way for judicial approval of any evidentiary expedition which on its own facts might seem to fall within that ill-defined limit. There are, I believe, grave dangers inseparably incidental to the precedent the court thus sets.

***

"No one can confidently predict how far today's decision actually goes. While it professes to stop short of a declaration 'that a court may authorize any challenged operation, no matter how major,' it clearly sanctions any judicially approved surgical operation which may be thought to be 'minor.' It furnishes no standard by which necessary differentiations between 'major' and 'minor' undertakings are to be achieved, nor any assistance to judges who must function in the no man's land in which they are to be made. In sum, it leaves to *ad hoc* determination, simply on the elastic and imprecise scale of reasonableness, the extent to which the arm of government may reach inside the human body. That, I fear, starts us down a slippery slope — on which there can be no stopping."

* * *

(The concurring opinion by Judge McGowan and the dissenting opinion by Judge Leventhal are deleted.)

* * *

COMMISSIONER OF CORRECTION V. MYERS

(Supreme Judicial Court of Massachusetts, 1979)
399 N.E. 2d 452

May a competent adult prisoner be forced to undergo dialysis treatments?

CHIEF JUSTICE HENNESSEY:

* * *

"...The defendant Kenneth Myers is an unmarried, mentally competent, twenty-four-year-old male. Since April 16, 1976, he has been serving several concurrent seven-to-ten-year sentences in Massachusetts correctional institutions....

"While in prison, the defendant developed a kidney condition diagnosed as chronic glomerulo-nephritis and uremia. When the kidney condition worsened, the defendant began receiving hemodialysis.... The treatment was administered three times a week in sessions of four hours' duration, with an additional hour spent connecting and disconnecting the machine.

"In addition to dialysis, the defendant received Kayexalate®, a medication that lowers the blood's potassium level. Kayexalate was normally prescribed only on weekends, the longest periods between regularly scheduled dialysis, to alleviate the risk of sudden death from cardiac arrest.... [T]he defendant could survive only three to five days if he refused both dialysis and Kayexalate, but he could survive ten to fifteeen days if he took the medication alone.

"For one year the defendant submitted to dialysis without significant complaint. However, on November 29, 1978, the defendant refused his regularly scheduled dialysis. He continued to refuse treatment the next day and, for a while, also refused the Kayexalate medication. Although efforts were made to persuade him to accept dialysis, there was no attempt to treat him without his consent. The defendant finally consented to dialysis on December 1, after the Commissioner had filed his complaint. However, the defendant did not indicate a willingness to continue dialysis in the future and, in fact, threatened to refuse treatment at any time.

"After the evidentiary hearing, the court concluded that the defendant's refusal of treatment had 'little to do with his disease, the nature or effects of the dialysis treatment, or the personal ramifications of continuing such treatment for the remainder of his life.' His refusal was also unrelated to any religious objection to the treatments. Nor did the defendant wish to die. Rather, the court found that 'Myers' refusal to take dialysis constitute(d) a form of protest against his placement in a medium, as opposed to a minimum, security prison.' As found by the court, this protest stemmed from the defendant's belief that continued hemodialysis weakened him and reduced his ability to defend himself against other inmates.

***

"...Doctor Chung testified that medical ethics demanded that everything possible be done to dialyze the defendant 'up to the point we cannot technically manage it.' Nonetheless, he admitted that he had never administered dialysis to an unwilling patient nor heard of others doing so and that it was not possible to use a general anesthetic to subdue a patient. Doctor Chung also testified that in the unlikely but conceivable event that the patient's struggling dislodged one of the needles connected to his arm, three to four minutes loss of blood could prove fatal. Nevertheless, the court found that employ-

ing a combination of mechanical and human restraints...would provide 'a feasible, if not completely risk-free, means of physically im-
mobilizing the recipient so that involuntary treatment could be
accomplished.'

***

"Myer's prognosis contrasts sharply with that of Saikewicz. Although Myer's kidney disease...could be technically classified as 'incurable,' it clearly was not life-threatening in the sense that his 'life
(would) soon, and inevitably, be extinguished' regardless of the treatment he received.... Consequently, the State's interest in the preservation of life is 'quite strong' in this instance....

"Notwithstanding the foregoing considerations, the State's interest in the preservation of life does not invariably control the right
to refuse treatment in cases of positive prognosis....

"Appropriately, the judge below focused on the magnitude of the
invasion occasioned by hemodialysis. We appraised that invasion as
'relatively slight,' when compared to that involved in an amputation
or in chemotherapy. We conclude, however, that the judge took too
narrow a view of the obtrusiveness of dialysis. Unlike the relatively
simply [sic] and risk-free treatment of supportive oral or intravenous
medications,dialysis exacts a significant price from Myers in return
for saving his life. In spite of the fact that dialysis does not require
the sacrifice of a limb or entail substantial pain, it is a relatively complex procedure, which requires considerable commitment and en-
durance from the patient who must undergo the treatment three
times a week.

"Taken together, the great deference accorded the State's interest
in the preservation of life...and the defendant's interest in avoiding
significant, nonconsensual invasions of his bodily integrity yield a
very close balance of interests. What tips that balance decisively in
the direction of authorizing treatment without consent is...the
State's interest in upholding orderly prison administration.

"Although the fact of the defendant's incarceration does not *per se*
divest him of his right to privacy and interest in bodily integrity..., it
does impose limitations on those constitutional rights in terms of the
State interests unique to the prison context.... Among the governmental interests recognized in a prison setting are the preservation
of internal order and discipline, the maintenance of institutional se-

curity, and the rehabilitation of prisoners.... The Commissioner invokes these State interests by arguing, first, that the maintenance of proper discipline and the supervision of inmates mandate an authority to administer life-saving medical treatment without consent and, second, that the State's failure to prevent Myer's death would present a serious threat to prison order and security, not only by generating a possibly 'explosive' reaction among other inmates, but also by encouraging them to attempt similar forms of coercion in order to attain illegitimate ends.

***

"The final State interests lending support to our authorization of compulsory medical treatment in this case are the interests in maintaining the ethical integrity of the medical profession and in permitting hospitals to care fully for patients under their control.... [T]here is no indication from expert testimony that medical ethics would support a failure to employ lifesaving procedures here where the traumatic cost to the patient is not inordinate and the prognosis is good....

***

"The order of the Superior Court compelling the defendant to submit to hemodialysis treatment and to take supportive medications, when those measures are necessary to maintain his life, is affirmed."

***

RUIZ V. ESTELLE

(U.S. District Court, 1980)
503 F. Supp. 1265

Are provisions for medical care in the Texas prison system unconstitutional?

JUDGE JUSTICE:

***

"Major problems pervade all aspects of the medical care provided by the TDC (Texas Department of Corrections) to its inmates.

The personnel providing routine medical care are often unqualified; they are also wholly insufficient in numbers and deficiently supervised. The meager medical facilities, inadequately equipped and poorly maintained, do not meet state licensing requirements. Medical procedures are unsound and faulty at all levels of care. Initial processing, sick call methods, and transfer practices are all unnecessarily cumbersome, inefficient, and life-threatening. Proper medical treatment and practice is often sacrificed to exaggerated concerns about security. Medical records are so poorly maintained, and the entries made therein are so incomplete and inaccurate, as to be either useless or harmful in the day-to-day provision of medical care and in the review of care previously provided. Finally, the entire medical care 'system' is marked by an absence of any organizational structure, plan, or written procedures for the delivery of medical care or for the instruction, supervision, and review of the personnel putatively providing it. These factors combine to produce a system that persistently and predictably fails adequately to provide for the legitimate medical needs of the prison population.

"The number of physicians providing medical care for TDC inmates is woefully inadequate. In 1974, the report of the Texas Legislature's Joint Committee on Prison Reform noted that, to meet the American Correctional Association standards for its then 17,000 inmates, TDC needed nineteen full-time physicians. TDC has never begun to approach this figure. During most of 1974, TDC employed only one full-time physician for the entire system. On several occasions since then, only two or three full-time doctors were actually present in the system. Some improvement has occurred in recent years; at the time of trial, with an inmate population of over 26,000, TDC employed the equivalent of 12.6 full-time physicians. These physicians were apportioned between the HUH, the Diagnositic Unit, and the seventeen-unit infirmaries. A total of twenty positions for physicians were authorized for the budget year beginning September 1, 1979, but TDC experienced difficulty in finding physicians to take the jobs. Even if these vacancies were all filled, the physician staffs at HUH and the Diagnostic Unit would still be grossly insufficient, and some units would continue to lack a full-time doctor. Correctional medical experts for both the plaintiff-intervenor and the defendants testified to an immediate, imperative necessity for more physicians, to meet adequately the authentic medical needs of TDC's inmate population.

"In consequence of the shortage of doctors, inmate patients are consistently treated by lay personnel. Important medical decisions relating to inmate patients are routinely left in the hands of non-physicians. Even at HUH (which primarily treats inmates for whom sufficient appropriate treatment cannot be provided at the unit level), patients frequently have been admitted, 'treated,' and discharged without ever being seen by a doctor. At the unit level, where medical supervision is even more sparse, medical assistants and inmate helpers are regularly entrusted to make crucial decisions concerning the screening, treatment, referral, and medication of inmate patients reporting infirmities.

***

"Recruitment and retention of doctors in the TDC system has proven extremely difficult. Physicians, generally in high demand throughout the free community, understandably have little incentive to work in prison surroundings, especially when it is obvious that their lot will be overwork and lack of adequate facilities, equipment, and auxiliary staff. The fact that most TDC units are located in relatively small rural communities further limits TDC's success in recruiting qualified physicians. In the face of such difficulties, Doctor Ralph Gray, TDC's medical director, has, on several occasions, employed doctors who were not licensed to practice in the general community. These included foreign-trained doctors who had not yet passed the necessary examinations to permit them to practice in Texas, and also recent medical school graduates who were awaiting examination results before beginning residencies. Several of the licensed physicians he succeeded in employing lacked relevant medical experience.

"An acutely grim and unwarranted lack of licensed nurses obtains in the TDC medical care system. At the time of trial, TDC was running the Huntsville Hospital with no registered nurses (RN's). The only RN's in the entire TDC system work in the women's units. This situation results, in part, from TDC's present policy of refusing to consider hiring female nurses to work at the male units. Since male nurses comprise only 1 percent of all RN's in the nation, this decision limits severely the pool from which TDC can attract applicants.

In spite of the recruitment difficulties imposed by the all-male policy, TDC was able to employ five male RN's and several male licensed vocational nurses (LVN's) at HUH during the years 1975-77. However, these nurses, who were apparently competent, well-trained, and conscientious, found conditions at HUH intolerable. By the end of 1977, all had relinquished their employment. One group, which resigned *en masse*, stated that they were prompted to take this action by the inadequacy of the physician staff, the absence of any formal procedures, and TDC's lack of commitment toward improving the level of care. The nurses in question, trained to observe appropriate limitations of their roles and aware of the need to defer certain decisions to physicians, experienced particular difficulty in dealing with the hospital administrator and the medical assistants (MA's). These functionaries did not share similar perceptions concerning the legitimate reach of the nurse's position, preferring instead that nurses and MA's perform tasks properly entrusted only to physicians. Rather than attempting to correct the unsolved practical and ethical problems which caused the loss of these sorely needed nurses, TDC administrators effectively decided to function altogether without licensed nurses and ceased to request budget authorizations for RN and LVN positions.

"TDC's failure even to attempt to employ RN's and LVN's in its hospital and unit infirmaries vividly demonstrates its virtual abdication of responsibility for the provision of adequate health care for its inmates. In the free world, HUH certainly would not be permitted to function as a hospital without the presence of RN's around the clock.

"Medical assistants (MA's) perform the vast bulk of medical care provided by civilians at TDC. TDC attempts to employ persons with military or civilian experience as medical technicians for these positions; however, neither this experience nor any character of state licensure or certification is absolutely required. Thus, of the MA's working at TDC at the time of the inspections by expert witnesses in 1976 and 1978, only one or two had medically related licenses of any kind. Some of the persons employed by TDC as MA's had no prior training as medical technicians nor any experience with direct patient care; the previous experience of others had ended many years before they went to work for TDC. TDC itself provides MA's with no medical training or instruction, since these individuals are expected to learn their trade on the job. Even if an MA desired to improve and expand his knowledge on a voluntary and independent basis, the lack of supervision by physicians and the absence of basic medical reference texts at the units would make this effort virtually impossible.

"Although most of the MA's are neither licensed, certified, nor trained to accomplish auxiliary health care functions at TDC facilities, they routinely perform procedures that properly should be undertaken by a registered nurse or physician. Nearly all initial screening decisions are made by MA's. They make the determination as to whether an inmate receives any treatment at all; if so, what medication to prescribe; when to hold the inmate for examination by a physician; and when to refer the inmate patient to HUH or John Sealy (Hospital). Thus, the typical inmate's access to health care is regulated from the outset by persons who would be qualified to perform only orderly-type functions at a free-world hospital. Furthermore, at the units MA's conduct sick call, diagnose ailments, prescribe and dispense medicine, and watch over inmates in solitary confinement. As previously alluded to, an almost total absence of supervision over the activities of the MA's by qualified medical personnel compounds the problems. TDC has no policy or procedure for regularly investigating the MA's performance of their duties, either through observation and supervision by physicians or by examination of medical records. This lack of oversight permits MA's constantly to make decisions and to take actions far beyond their capabilities.

* * *

"Through fiscal year 1979, TDC made no provision for MA's to be on duty at its infirmaries on a twenty-four-hour basis, and only inmate nurses have been present at these facilities during the night. Both witnesses for the defendants and the plaintiffs agreed that the presence of civilian medical personnel at the infirmaries is essential at all times, since the evils inherent in a situation where inmates are responsible for the provision of medical care...are magnified when they are the only medical personnel on duty. Moreover, the medical crises of inmates which arise during night hours are often of an emergency nature, junctures which demand immediate and skilled medical treatment by qualified personnel....

* * *

"An inmate assigned to work in TDC's medical departments is not required to have any specific qualifications. Once assigned to the medical department, an inmate is provided little formal training of any kind, it being expected that he will learn his tasks by following and observing an experienced inmate nurse. Thus, even if such an inmate's duties were restricted to orderly work his training would be inadequate. The evidence revealed, however, that such inmates regularly perform procedures for which they are not qualified. These procedures have included administering intravenous injections to inmates, performing Pap tests, dispensing drugs without the supervision of an RN or physician, suturing lacerations, and providing other emergency care. Testimony has shown that inmate nurses often perform x-ray photography, conduct and interpret eye examinations, administer oral anesthesia, lance boils, and insert sutures. A few inmate nurses have regularly engaged in setting and casting broken bones, and one sutured heel tendons and performed fingertip amputation.

"Inmate nurses have also been instructed or permitted to make entries in their patient's charts. Deliberate falsifications in the charts are often made by those inmates (e.g. patients' liquid inputs and outputs have been improperly charted; spurious temperature readings have been inserted; and fictitious administrations of medications have been shown)....

* * *

"While inmate nurses all too often improperly undertake treatment functions for which they are unqualified, the record reveals the irony that they have been reluctant to perform certain basic custodial duties. Grievous neglect of the personal care of the patients at the HUH have resulted. Examples are numerous: on many occasions, routine preoperative enemas and urinalyses were not performed on time; urine bags were allowed to overflow (particularly on Monday morning, when no RN had been in the hospital all weekend); urine collections for urinalyses were either not accomplished or the specimens were not refrigerated, thus making them useless; intravenous solutions were allowed to run dry; bandages were not changed on time; incontinent inmates were allowed to lie in their own feces or urine for long periods; and inadequate hygienic care was administered to invalid patients generally. Decubitus ulcers (bedsores) were frequent among bedridden patients as a result of the inattentive nursing.

***

"Each TDC unit has its own infirmary, supposedly equipped in such manner as to enable the unit medical staff to cope with the everyday minor ailments of inmates, to diagnose and determine the appropriate level of treatment for more serious medical problems, to render critical emergency care, and to arrange for the expeditious transportation of emergency cases to a hospital. The results of TDC's severe overcrowding are also found here. Too many inmates are assigned to each unit for the infirmaries to serve these purposes effectively, since the exiguity of the examining rooms, office spaces, and beds in these facilities fall far short of meeting the demands placed upon them. At least as late as the 1978 re-inspections by the expert witnesses who testified, suitable emergency equipment, laboratory equipment, and physical therapy facilities were still wanting.

"The lack of reliable emergency transportation from the units to HUH, John Sealy [Hospital], or community hospitals have been manifested repeatedly. On many occasions, breakdowns of ambulance equipment and related difficulties have resulted in inordinate delays in the transfer of emergency patients to hospitals. To some extent, improved equipment has been obtained, but a reliable alternative arrangement for ambulance service in the event of an ambulance breakdown is not available at every unit. Furthermore, most TDC ambulances are deficient of certain necessary equipment and competently trained paramedical personnel to operate them.

"It is highly questionable whether TDC's 'hospital' at Huntsville can be accurately labeled as such. HUH violates state hospital licensing requirements and lost its Texas Hospital Association (THA) accreditation many years ago. It is obvious, then, that THA would not permit a comparable facility serving free-world patients to operate in Texas. Notwithstanding the full, definite and longstanding knowledge of its gross inadequacies by TDC's highest officials, HUH has been used as the system's primary health care facility for many years. Antiquated, poorly designed, unacceptably equipped, and deficiently maintained HUH is, in addition, extremely overcrowded....

"Witnesses from both sides agreed that the facility was old, in disrepair, inadequately staffed, insufficiently organized and lacking in the most basic equipment. The most shocking deficiency is the continued absence of adequate fire-fighting equipment or safe means of exit from the hospital in case of fire. With chilling indifference, TDC officials routinely permit seriously ill or injured inmates, a substantial number of whom are bedridden, to be placed in this facility that, since 1974, has been known to violate fire safety standards.

***

"The shortage of pharmaceutical professionals has led to the use of medical assistants, security officers, and even inmates to staff the pill rooms. These persons regularly perform duties that, in a free-world pharmacy, could only be handled by a licensed pharmacist. Unit medical assistants do not possess the necessary pharmaceutical training and lack the requisite qualifications to operate a pharmacy without the supervision of a trained, licensed pharmacist. The security officers who are on duty in many of the unit pill rooms have even less training and are more unqualified to handle medicines; furthermore, their deployment as pharmaceutical assistants depletes the already meager ranks of personnel performing true security functions. Even more egregious is the use of inmates to dispense medications, a practice universally condemned by the expert witnesses who testified. TDC claims to have taken steps to eliminate inmates from functioning in the pill room; but at the time of trial, this objective has not been achieved.

***

"An additional matter causing perturbation to the expert witnesses were unit pharmaceutical operations, where the tendency of TDC personnel to overmedicate inmates manifested itself most obviously. On a number of occasions, they testified, inmates were given larger doses of medication than were warranted, particularly in instances involving such powerful and potentially dangerous drugs as Thorazine®. Additionally, medical personnel have shaken off importunate inmates voicing medical complaints by prescribing for the latter medically uncalled-for drugs. The expert witnesses testified that this practice has negative implications for the quality of medical care, in that it functions as a substitute for careful diagnosis and evaluation of inmate complaints, results in inappropriate treatment for serious conditions, and increases the possibilities of drug abuse among the inmate population. Indeed, among the drugs routinely dispensed at TDC have been large quantities of behavior-altering drugs with a high potential for abuse....

***

"...[I]solated incidents of medical malpractice, carelessness, or indifference to inmate medical needs by guards or administrators, or occasional mistakes in processing or classifying an inmate patient, do not give rise to claims of constitutional proportion. However, a pattern of such occurrences extending over a period of time or the existence of systemic deficiencies which will inevitably lead to unnecessary pain and distress constitute proof of deliberate indifference to the medical needs of inmates.

"The record in the instant case is replete with examples of such deliberate indifference, manifested by improper handling of individual cases and by failure to correct persistent, systematic deficiencies. These faults, well known to the defendants, have resulted in a medical system so inadequate for the inmates needs that their sufferings are inevitably increased and prolonged. The individual examples ...are not, as characterized by the defendants, merely a few isolated incidents, or 'horror stories.' Instead, they establish a continuous pattern of harmful, inadequate medical treatment, which manifests itself frequently and injuriously in the lives of inmate patients.

***

"On the basis of the evidence presented, and the applicable law, it becomes clear that TDC's medical care system fails to comply with the Eighth Amendment to the Constitution [the cruel and unusual punishment clause].* To remedy these egregious circumstances, TDC will be required to increase staffing for all medical personnel, to restrict the use of inmates to perform medical and pharmacological functions, to improve unit infirmary facilities, and either to substantially renovate HUH or downgrade it to an infirmary. In addition, it will be mandated that TDC establish diagnostic and sick-call procedures which eliminate non-medical interferences with

---

*"In contrast to the rest of TDC's medical facilities, conditions at the John Sealy Hospital do meet the requirements of the Constitution."

the provision of medical care, as well as medically sound procedures for making job assignments. Finally, the deficiencies in pharmaceutical operations, record-keeping and overall organization of medical care delivery services, noted herein, must be remedied."

***

JACKSON V. INDIANA

(U.S. Supreme Court, 1972)
406 U.S. 715

May an incompetent who will never become competent be indefinitely committed to an institution solely on account of lack of capacity to stand trial?

JUSTICE BLACKMAN:

***

"Petitioner, Theon Jackson, is a mentally defective deaf mute with a mental level of a pre-school child. He cannot read, write, or otherwise communicate except through limited sign language. In May 1968, at age 27, he was charged...with separate robberies of two women.... The first involved property (a purse and its contents) of the value of four dollars. The second concerned five dollars in money....

"As the statute requires, the court appointed two psychiatrists to examine Jackson. A competency hearing was subsequently held at which petitioner was represented by counsel. The court received the examining doctor's joint written report and oral testimony from them and from a deaf-school interpreter through whom they had attempted to communicate with petitioner. The report concluded that Jackson's almost non-existent communication skill, together with his lack of hearing and his mental deficiency, left him unable to understand the nature of the charges against him or to participate in his defense. One doctor testified that it was extremely unlikely that petitioner could ever learn to read or write and questioned whether petitioner even had the ability to develop any proficiency in sign language. He believed that the interpreter had not been able to communicate with petitioner to any great extent and testified that petitioner's 'prognosis appears rather dim.' The other doctor testified that even if Jackson were not a deaf mute, he would be incompetent to stand trial, and doubted whether petitioner had sufficient intelligence ever to develop the necessary communications skills. The interpreter testified that Indiana had no facilities that could help someone as badly off as Jackson to learn minimal communication skills.

"On this evidence, the trial court found that Jackson 'lack[ed] comprehension sufficient to make his defense,' section 9-1706a, and ordered him committed to the Indiana Department of Mental Health until such time as that Department should certify to the court that 'the defendant is sane.'

"Petitioner's counsel then filed a motion for a new trial, contending that there was no evidence that Jackson was 'insane,' or that he would ever attain a status which the court might regard as 'sane' in the sense of competency to stand trial. Counsel argued that Jackson's commitment under these circumstances amounted to a 'life sentence' without his ever having been convicted of a crime, and that the commitment therefore deprived Jackson of his Fourteenth Amendment rights to due process and equal protection....

"For the reasons set forth below, we conclude that, on the record before us, Indiana cannot constitutionally commit the petitioner for an indefinite period simply on account of his incompetency to stand trial on the charges filed against him. Accordingly, we reverse.

* * *

"Because the evidence established little likelihood of improvement in petitioner's condition, he argues that commitment under section 9-1706a in his case amounted to a commitment for life. This deprived him of equal protection, he contends, because, absent the criminal charges pending against him, the State would have had to proceed under other statutes generally applicable to all other citizens: either the commitment procedures for feeble-minded persons, or those for mentally ill persons. He argues that under these other statutes (1) the decision whether to commit would have been made according to a different standard, (2) if commitment were warranted, applicable standards of release would have been more lenient, (3) if committed under section 22-1907, he could have been assigned to a special institution affording appropriate care, and (4) he would have been entitled to certain privileges not now available to him.

* * *

"Respondent argues, however, that because the record fails to establish affirmatively that Jackson will never improve, his commitment 'until sane' is not really an indeterminate one. It is only temporary, pending possible change in his condition. Thus, presumably, it cannot be judged against commitments under other state statutes that are truly indeterminate. The State relies on the lack of 'exactitude' with which psychiatry can predict the future course of mental illness....

"Were the State's factual premise that Jackson's commitment is only temporary a valid one, this might well be a different case. But the record does not support that premise. One of the doctors testified that in his view Jackson would be unable to acquire substantially improved communication skills that would be necessary for him to participate in any defense. The prognosis for petitioner's developing such skills, he testified, appeared 'rather dim.' In answer to a question whether Jackson would ever be able to comprehend the charges or participate in his defense, even after commitment and treatment, the doctor said, 'I doubt it, I don't believe so.' The other psychiatrist testified that even if Jackson were able to develop such skills, he would still be unable to comprehend the proceedings or aid counsel due to his mental deficiency. The interpreter, a supervising teacher at the state school for the deaf, said that he would not be able to serve as an interpreter for Jackson or aid him in participating in a trial, and that the State had no facilities that could, 'after a length of time' aid Jackson in so participating. The court also heard petitioner's mother testify that Jackson already had undergone rudimentary outpatient training in communications skills from the deaf and dumb school in Indianapolis over a period of three years without noticeable success. There is nothing in the record that even points to any possibility that Jackson's present condition can be remedied at any future time.

* * *

"We note also that neither the Indiana statute nor state practice makes the likelihood of the defendant's improvement a relevant factor. The State did not seek to make any such showing, and the record clearly establishes that the chances of Jackson's ever meeting the competency standards of section 9-1706a are at best minimal, if not nonexistent. The record also rebuts any contention that the commitment could contribute to Jackson's improvement. Jackson's section 9-1706a commitment is permanent in practical effect.

"We therefore must turn to the question whether, because of the pendency of the crimnal charges that triggered the State's invocation of section 9-1706a, Jackson was deprived of substantial rights to which he would have been entitled under either of the other two state commitment statutes. *Baxstrom* held that the State cannot withhold from a few the procedural protections or the substantive requirements for commitment that are available to all others. In this case, commitment procedures under all three statutes appear substantially similar: notice, examination by two doctors, and a full judicial hearing at which the individual is represented by counsel and can cross-examine witnesses and introduce evidence. Under each of the three statutes, the commitment determination is made by the court alone, and appellate review is available.

"In contrast, however, what the State must show to commit a defendant under section 9-1706a, and the circumstances under which an individual so committed may be released, are substantially different from the standards under the other two statutes.

"Under section 9-1706a, the State needed to show only Jackson's inability to stand trial. We are unable to say that, on the record before us, Indiana could have civilly committed him as mentally ill under section 22-1209 or committed him as feeble-minded under section 22-1907. The former requires at least (1) a showing of mental illness and (2) a showing that the individual is in need of 'care, treatment, training or detention....' Whether Jackson's mental deficiency would meet the first test is unclear; neither examining physician addressed himself to this. Furthermore, it is problematical whether commitment for 'treatment' or 'training' would be appropriate since the record establishes that none is available for Jackson's condition at any state institution. The record also fails to establish that Jackson is in need of custodial care or 'detention.' He has been employed at times, and there is no evidence that the care he long received at home has become inadequate. The statute appears to require an independent showing of dangerousness... Insofar as it may require such a showing, the pending criminal charges are insufficient to establish it, and no other supporting evidence was introduced....

"More important, an individual committed as feeble-minded is eligible for release when his condition 'justifies it'...and an individual civilly committed as mentally ill when the 'superintendent or administrator shall discharge such person *or*[when] cured of such illness,.... Thus, in either case release is appropriate when the individual no longer requires the custodial care or treatment or detention that occasioned the commitment, or when the department of mental health believes release would be in his best interests. The evidence available concerning Jackson's past employment and home care strongly suggests that under these standards he might be eligible for release at almost any time, even if he did not improve. On the other hand, by the terms of his present section 9-1706a commitment, he will not be entitled to release at all, absent an unlikely substantial change for the better in his condition.

***

"As we noted above, we cannot conclude that pending criminal charges provide greater justification for different treatment than conviction and sentence. Consequently, we hold that by subjecting Jackson to a more lenient commitment standard and to a more stringent standard of release than those generally applicable to all others not charged with offenses, and by thus condemning him in effect to permanent institutionalization,...Indiana deprived petitioner of equal protection of the laws under the Fourteenth Amendment.

***

"It is clear that Jackson's commitment rests on proceedings that did not purport to bring into play, indeed did not even consider relevant, any of the articulated bases for exercise of Indiana's power of indefinite commitment. The state statutes contain at least two alternative methods for invoking this power. But Jackson was not afforded any 'formal commitment procedings addressed to [his] ability to function in society,' or to society's interest in his restraint, or to the State's ability to aid him in attaining competency through custodial care or compulsory treatment, the ostensible purpose of the commitment. At the least, due process requires that the nature and duration of commitment bear some reasonable relation to the purpose for which the individual is committed.

"We hold, consequently, that a person charged by a State with a criminal offense who is committed solely on account of his incapacity to proceed to trial cannot be held more than the reasonable period of time necessary to determine whether there is a substantial probability that he will attain that capacity in the foreseeable future. If it is determined that this is not the case, then the State must either institute the customary civil commitment proceeding that would be required to commit indefinitely any other citizen, or release the defendant. Furthermore, even if it is determined that the defendant probably soon will be able to stand trial, his continued commitment must be justified by progress toward that goal. In light of differing state facilities and procedures and a lack of evidence in this record, we do not think it appropriate for us to attempt to prescribe arbitrary time limits. We note, however, that petitioner Jackson has now been confined for three-and-one-half years on a record that sufficiently establishes the lack of a substantial probability that he will ever be able to participate fully in a trial.

***

"Reversed and remanded."

(Mr. Justice Powell and Mr. Justice Rehnquist took no part in the consideration or decision of this case.)

WINTERS V. MILLER

(U.S. Court of Appeals, Second Circuit, 1971)
446 F. 2d 65

May a woman in a mental institution who has not been found incompetent be forced to undergo medical treatments against her wishes and her religious beliefs?

JUDGE JOSEPH SMITH:

***

"Miss Miriam Winters is a 59-year-old spinster who has been supported under public assistance for over 10 years. For several years she has lived in a hotel in Brooklyn, New York and had created some difficulty there because of her constant demands that she be given a room with a private bath and because of her alleged failure to maintain a proper state of personal cleanliness.

"In early 1967, she was told by her welfare case worker that she could obtain a room with a private bath with the approval of a physician or a psychiatrist. Accordingly, at her request, she was seen by Doctor Robert Reich, a psychiatric consultant to the Department of Welfare. Following this examination, Miss Winters was told that she would be given a room with a private bath if she would move to the King Edward Hotel in Manhattan, which she agreed to do, and in mid-April she took up residence there. On May 2, 1968 when Miss Winters attempted to pay her rent for that month she was told by the hotel management that she could not continue to occupy the room she was in but would have to move to another room in the same hotel. This she refused to do, and as a result, the hotel management summoned the police, and she was taken by them to Bellvue Hospital where she was involuntarily admitted pursuant to section 78(1) of the New York Mental Hygiene Law.... On May 7, 1968 appellant was examined by two staff psychiatrists at Bellvue who certified her need for care pursuant to section 72(1) of the New York Mental Hygiene Law which provides for commitment for up to 60 days upon the filing of a 'two physician certificate.'

"For 10 years prior to her admission to Bellvue, Miss Winters had been a practicing Christian Scientist. When she was admitted, she refused to allow a doctor to take her blood pressure, stating to him that she was a Christian Scientist, and the Bellvue records contain several references to this fact, indicating that the hospital clearly had notice of her religious beliefs. In spite of this, however, and over her continued objections she was given medication (for the most part rather heavy doses of tranquilizers, both orally and intramuscularly) continually from the time of her admission until she was discharged on June 18, 1968. On May 13, 1968 she was transferred from Bellvue to the Central Islip State Hospital on Long Island. Again the record clearly indicates that she brought her objections to physical medication to the attention of the hospital staff, but her protests were ignored.

"The primary question raised in this appeal is whether appellant's constitutional rights were violated when she was given medical treatment over her objections, which were religious in nature....

***

"It is clear and appellees concede that if we were dealing here with an ordinary patient suffering from a physical ailment, the hospital authorities would have no right to impose compulsory medical treatment against the patient's will and, indeed, that to do so would constitute a common law assault and battery. The question then becomes at what point, if at all, does the patient suffering from a mental illness lose the rights he would otherwise enjoy in this regard?

"The court below was apparently of the view that *any* patient alleged to be suffering from a mental illness of *any* kind (even those confined under the 'emergency' provisions of section 78(1) where the allegations of mental illness need not be made by a physician) loses the right to make a decision on whether or not to accept treatment. Judge Travis reasoned as follows: 'In mental cases, the public interest in treating and caring for patients is greater than the public interest in the cases of physical illness. Most patients who are physically ill will be able to determine that they need treatment and, when informed by their physicians, will be able to make a reasoned decision as to the type of treatment to which they wish to subject themselves. But a mental patient, because of the nature of his illness, may be unable either to seek appropriate treatment or to determine what treatment to allow. For the physically ill person, where there are no dependent children or communicable disease involved, the danger from a refusal on religious or any other grounds to allow a particular type of treatment may be that the patient will die. Only the patient and his immediate family are likely to be aggrieved or injured as a result. On the other hand, where the mental patient is not properly treated, the condition may progressively worsen, and the patient may become a public burden and expense. Badly needed beds in mental hospitals may be occupied by those (few or many) who refuse treatment which competent and expert medical practitioners prescribe. Where the proposed treatment is conducive or necessary for the cure or amelioration of mental illness, the failure to provide it would be a step backward in the history of mental hygiene....'

* * *

"...While it may be true that the state could validly undertake to treat Miss Winters if it did stand in a *parens patriae* relationship to her and such a relationship may be created if and when a person is found legally incompetent, there was never any effort on the part of appellees to secure such a judicial determination of incompetency before proceeding to treat Miss Winters in the way they thought would be 'best' for her. As appellant points out, even if there is some way to find the kind of compelling state interest required to override the First Amendment, there clearly was not a compelling interest in so summarily forcing her to do so. Regular hearings of the New York Supreme Court are held in Bellvue Hospital every Tuesday morning. Plaintiff was admitted on Thursday evening. If appellees had respected her wishes for only four days, they could have brought her before the court for judicial resolution of the issue. At this hearing the appellant might have been able to persuade the court that she was not mentally ill. Or the court might have found that other alternatives would suffice. Under our Constitution there is no procedural right more fundamental than the right of the citizen, except in extraordinary circumstances, to tell his side of the story to an impartial tribunal....

"Having concluded, therefore, that the appellant has stated a claim on which relief may be granted, we remand the case to the district court with instructions that it proceed to trial on the merits."

* * *

JUDGE MOORE DISSENTING IN PART:

* * *

"...[T]he majority in my judgement is not correct in its conclusions that plaintiff was in anyway unjustifiably denied her constitutional rights.

"After asserting, in effect, that there is no basis here for finding Miss Winters to be possibly harmful to herself and others, the majority suggests that 'it may be true that the state could validly undertake to treat Miss Winters if it did stand in a *parens patriae* relationship to her' and that 'such a relationship may be created if and when a person is found *legally* incompetent,' and not be a proceeding under sections 72(1) or 78(1).

"Does the majority mean by this that a person who is deemed to be potentially harmful to others could not, even in an emergency situation, be given appropriate drugs to reduce the likelihood of such anti-social conduct in the absence of an adversary judicial determination of incompetence? In the face of danger to herself and others, must Bellvue's harried medical staff seek out a judge whenever the police present them with a person whose mental condition requires that she receive tranquilizers or other drugs to protect herself and others, or do they mean that a person can be given drugs against his stated religious convictions in at least some circumstances where the patient has not been declared legally incompetent by judicial adversary determination?

"I disagree in any event with the majority's implicit conclusion that...the treating doctors were not justified in concluding that the medical treatment administered was not in the best interests of the patient and, on the contrary, would hold that this determination being valid, justified the medical care given Miss Winters. The Millsian distinction between instances of harm to others and instances of harm solely to self, relied on by the majority, would seem rarely if ever to be relevant in actuality because others are affected by virtually any action which an individual takes or fails to take. Thus, while Miss Winters might not have been likely to perpetuate a violent attack on her fellow patients had she not received the tranquilizers here involved, the very conduct which led to her admission, if repeated in the ward, might well have been disruptive to the recovery of others in her ward, who themselves may have been suffering from psychological defects. Second, even if no one other than Miss Winters would have been directly aided by the treatment for the condition for which she was admitted, as Judge Travis pointed out in his opinion below, if mentally ill persons are not accorded proper treatment, their 'condition may progressively worsen, and the patient may become a public burden and expense.'

"More fundamentally, I believe that a section 78(1) admission, as well as a two-physician admission under section 72(1), constitutes a quasi-judicial determination under state law authorizing medical care of an individual, notwithstanding her lack of consent thereto...."

* * *

ROGERS V. OKIN

(U.S. District Court, 1979)
478 F. Supp. 1942

Do institutionalized mental patients have a right to refuse medication?

JUDGE TAURO:

***

"Plaintiffs allege that the defendants have impermissibly followed a policy of forcibly medicating committed mental patients, and that such policy has denied them their constitutionally protected right to refuse treatment. Although plaintiffs urge this court to recognize a right to refuse treatment, they do not maintain that such a right is absolute. They acknowledge that in emergencies it must yield to the state's interest in medicating.

"Defendants proffer a three-pronged defense to plaintiffs' allegations. First, they maintain that a committed mental patient is *per se* incompetent to decide whether or not to receive treatment. Second, they deny that any patient was forcibly medicated except in circumstances amounting to at least a psychiatric emergency. Third, they assert that committed mental patients, whether voluntary or involuntary, have no constitutional right to refuse treatment in any situation — emergency or non-emergency.

***

"A pivotal issue dividing the parties in this case is the competency of mental patients to decide rationally whether or not to receive treatment....

***

"The weight of evidence persuades this court that, although committed mental patients do suffer at least some impairment of their relationship to reality, most are able to appreciate the benefits, risks, and discomfort that may reasonably be expected from receiving psychotropic medication. This is particularly true for patients who have experienced such medication and, therefore, have some basis for assessing comparative advantages and disadvantages. Indeed, a fundamental concept for treating the mentally ill is the establishment of a therapeutic alliance between psychiatrist and patient. Implicit in such an alliance is an understanding and acceptance by the patient of a prescribed treatment program.

"Moreover, defendant's position that commitment *per se* demonstrates the incompetence of a mental patient to decide treatment questions is at odds with...[state laws and regulations]. These provisions state unequivocally that, although committed, a mental patient is nonetheless presumed competent to manage his affairs, dispose of property, carry on a licensed profession, and even to vote. That presumption of competency prevails unless and until there has been an adjudication of incompetency by a court, following notice and hearing....

"To be sure, these regulatory provisions do not expressly grant mental patients a right to refuse treatment, except with respect to electrical shock and lobotomy. But...regulations do recognize in absolute terms the competence of committed persons to manage their affairs and participate in a variety of challenging activities. That recognition tilts the scales in favor of presuming, as well, the competence of a committed mental patient to make treatment decisions, absent an adjudication to the contrary.

* * *

"This court concludes...that committed mental patients are presumed competent to make decisions with respect to their treatment in non-emergencies. Given an adjudication of incompetence, a guardian may exercise for and on behalf of a committed mental patient any right she may have to make treatment decisions in a non-emergency.

"...[T]he parties agree that forced medication is permissible in an emergency situation. They disagree, however, as to what circumstances amount to an emergency situation justifying such treatment.

* * *

"The court recognizes that varying degrees of crisis may typify the average day on a ward of any mental institution. Patient behavior can be challenging, to say the least. Attendant staff must respond to such behavior in a manner that is appropriate, reasonable and adequate. Given circumstances creating a substantial likelihood of physical harm to the patient or others, the Commonwealth, acting through hospital staff, may respond so as to ensure safety in the hospital community. The state's *parens patriae* interest in protecting the safety of the people extends to the microcosm world of the hospital, as well as the community at large.

***

"This court holds, therefore, that a committed mental patient may be forcibly medicated in an emergency situation in which a failure to do so would result in a substantial likelihood of physical harm to that patient, other patients, or to staff members of the institution.

"Given the uncontested right of the state to impose treatment without informed consent in an emergency, the court must now decide whether the state has a comparable right in a non-emergency. Because the state contends that the status of voluntary and involuntary patients is substantively different, their rights will be considered separately.

***

"The prime purpose of any hospital is to treat. Boston State is no exception. In the case of an involuntarily committed patient, Boston State has a duty to provide treatment. Stated another way, the involuntarily committed patient has a right to receive treatment. The question here is whether the hospital's duty to provide necessary treatment carries with it an implicit right to impose such treatment contrary to a patient's expressed wishes. In considering this question, it is important to have in mind that plaintiffs do not assert a right to refuse all treatment at all times. Their prime contention is that committed patients have a right not to be forcibly injected with psychotropic medication in a non-emergency situation, or where there are less drastic or less invasive alternatives available.

"This court has already found that psychotropic medications are powerful and potentially mind-altering drugs.... Plaintiffs argue that the forcible injection, without informed consent, of such medication violates a patient's constitutional right to privacy....

***

"The defendants concede that a right to privacy may include 'the interest in independence in making certain kinds of important decisions....' But, they argue that plaintiffs' interest in refusing treatment in a mental institution setting is not a right fundamental to concepts of ordered liberty traditionally recognized and protected by the Supreme Court.

"The defendant's position does not give due regard to the plight of a patient who has been committed to a state mental institution. We know that the committed mental patient has been quarantined from home, family and society, not for adjudged criminal activity, but because of sickness — mental illness.

* * *

"At final argument, the Commonwealth conceded that a committed patient would have the right to sell his home, but maintained that the patient has no rights with respect to what treatment to receive, if any, in a non-emergency situation. Common sense dictates a contrary conclusion, however. Certainly the right to dispose of one's property, and the corollary right to protect and hold such property, are fundamental to any concept of ordered liberty.... But, such rights pale in comparison to the intimate decision as to whether to accept or refuse psychotropic medication — medication that may or may not make the patient better, and that may or may not cause unpleasant and unwanted side effects. The right to make such a decision is basic to any right of privacy.

"The concept of a right of privacy also embodies First Amendment concerns. It is clear from the evidence in this case that psychotropic medication has the potential to affect and change a patient's mood, attitude and capacity to think. Such effects may well be considered by the medical profession as positive steps on the road to recovery and eventual release from the hospital. But, the validity of psychotropic drugs as a reasonable course of medical treatment is not the core issue here. At stake is the more fundamental question as to whether the state may impose once again on the privacy of a person, already deprived of freedom through commitment, by forcibly injecting mind-altering drugs into his system in a non-emergency situation.

* * *

"The First Amendment protects the communication of ideas. That protected right of communication presupposes a capacity to produce ideas. As a practical matter, therefore, the power to produce ideas is fundamental to our cherished right to communicate and is entitled to comparable constitutional protection. Whatever powers the Constitution has granted our government, involuntary mind control is not one of them, absent extraordinary circumstances. The fact that mind control takes place in a mental institution in the form of medically sound treatment of mental disease is not, itself, an extraordinary circumstance warranting an unsanctioned intrusion on the integrity of a human being. The patient is in an institution only because he is unable to function safely in society, and so there is a public interest in civil commitment. The state may not involuntarily commit a person merely because of bizarre or unorthodox behavior.

"The concept of a therapeutic alliance between doctor and patient presumes a communication of information as to the pros and cons of a particular treatment program. The committed patient has a right to be wrong in his analysis of that information — a right to be unwise — as long as the consequences of such error do not pose a danger of physical harm to himself, fellow patients or hospital staff. And so, while the state may have an obligation to make treatment available, and a legitimate interest in providing such treatment, a competent patient has a fundamental right to decide to be left alone, absent an emergency situation.

"Defendants argue that voluntary patients may not refuse medication, even in non-emergencies, and still remain at the Hospital. Their position is that patients volunteering for commitment implicitly agree to accept the Hospital's treatment program and may not second-guess the institution staff by picking and choosing the type of medication to be used. Basically, the defendants argue a contract theory that would supersede and amount to a waiver of any supposed right of refusal.

"All voluntary patients sign an appliction that states: 'I understand that during my hospitalization and any after care, I will be given care and treatment which may include the injection of medicines....'

"Clearly, parties competent to contract may not accept provisions of the bargain they favor and then reject those they wish to avoid. But, such a truth serves only to raise the question presented here, not answer it. One remedy for the unhappy voluntary patient is clear, leaving the hospital. But procedures for doing so require a hiatus of three days' notice from the patient to the hospital superintendent.... The issue, therefore, is really twofold: (1) what is the voluntary patient's right to refuse treatment from the time of departure from the hospital; and (2) even prior to notice, or absent notice, does the voluntary patient have a constitutional right to refuse treatment despite any contractual obligation that may have been established by the voluntary commitment?

"This court holds that the voluntary patient has the same right to refuse treatment in a non-emergency as does the involuntary patient, and that on the facts of this case there has been no waiver of such right.

***

"In order for a court to find a waiver of a right to refuse, the evidence must be clear that the patient understood such a right existed and then elected knowingly and voluntarily to waive such a right. The language proffered by the defendants contains neither element. The Commonwealth drafted the language in the application and the defendants, as agents of the Commonwealth, must bear the burden of its inadequacy.

"The Supreme Court has long recognized that fundamental rights are not absolute, but may be subordinated to compelling state interests.... The state has no such compelling interest here.

***

"That the state may forcibly medicate a committed patient given an emergency that threatens the physical safety of patients and staff—the institutional community—is not at issue. Such action is necessary to protect the members of that community.... Given a non-emergency, however, it is an unreasonable invasion of privacy, and an affront to basic concept of human dignity, to permit forced injection of a mind-altering drug into the buttocks of a competent patient unwilling to give informed consent. That type of treatment is not necessary to protect the general public, since the patient has already been quarantined by commitment. Of course, there being no emergency, the hospital community is in no danger.

"The only purpose, therefore, of forced medication, in a non-emergency, is to help the patient. The desire to help the patient is a laudable if not noble goal. But a basic premise of the right to privacy is the freedom to decide whether we want to be helped, or whether we want to be left alone. It takes a grave set of circumstances to abrogate that right. That a non-emergency injection in the buttocks may be therapeutic does not constitute such a circumstance.

* * *

"There are alternative methods of treating mental patients, though some may be slower and less effective than psychotropic medication. As has been noted, plaintiffs' primary objection is to the forced injection of psychotropic medication. Given the alternatives available in non-emergencies, subjecting a patient to the humiliation of being disrobed and then injected with drugs powerful enough to immobilize both body and mind is totally unreasonable by any standard....

"Aside from the proffered state interests in forced medication, the defendants also resist recognizing a right to refuse by challenging the efficacy of a regime of informed consent. The defendants' crystal ball foretells a tale of gloom if the standards imposed by this court's temporary restraining order (TRO) are made permanent. But, their prediction is not borne out by the experience of that order. Although Doctor Gill expressed concern as to the impact of the TRO on effective treatment, he could identify only 12 patients out of 1,000 who refused their medication for prolonged periods between May 1, 1975 and June 23, 1977 — and most of those changed their minds within a few days.

"None of these patients were transferrd to a more secure institutional setting because of behavior problems.

"Should the TRO be made permanent, defendants foresee institutional settings becoming mere warehouses, characterized by increases in violence, patient apathy, length of stays and administrative problems. The evidence in this case, however, demonstrates that such a gloomy forecast is more dramatic than factual.

* * *

"In an *amicus* brief, the Massachusetts Psychiatric Society argues: 'If forbidden to use certain standard, effective modalities, they [hospital staffs] will be caught in the situation of having a legal obligation which they cannot carry out.'

"...That argument suffers from a faulty premise. The state has a duty to make treatment available. It has no duty to impose treatment on a competent involuntary patient who prefers to refuse medication, regardless of its potential benefit.

"In analyzing defendants' prediction of doom should the TRO be made permanent, it is helpful to recall the testimony of the defendants and most of their expert witnesses, to the effect that they would respect a patient's preference to refuse treatment, absent an emergency situation. In other words, although not conceding a patient's legal right to refuse treatment, the professional's practice is to honor the refusal, except in an emergency. That testimony is inconsistent with a prediction of a chaotic institutional atmosphere if patients' wishes to refuse medication are honored. Certainly the expressed attitude of these interested professionals demonstrates that respecting and abiding by a competent mental patient's wishes concerning medication would not undermine the ethical integrity of the medical profession.

"The Commonwealth does have a legitimate interest in decreasing the number of patients hospitalized, as well as the length of their stays. One need only to be alive to be aware that the costs of illness, mental and physical, are soaring. There may well be additional administrative expense and burden attached to recognizing a competent inpatient's right to refuse treatment. Stated another way, it might be less expensive for the state to deny, rather than recognize, such a right. But, factors of convenience and cost have long been regarded as inadequate justifications, standing alone, for a state's failure to recognize and respect constitutionally protected rights....

"One basic theme that seems to thread its way through most of defendant's arguments is that a federal court has no business second-guessing a treatment decision of a hospital staff person. This contention is like saying that once there is confinement in prison there can be no judicial scrutiny as to the conditions of confinement....

* * *

"The defendants are enjoined from forcibly medicating committed mental patients, voluntary or involuntary, except in emergency circumstances in which a failure to do so would bring about a substantial likelihood of physical harm to the patient or others. An order will issue."

* * *

QUESTIONS

1. Is a lack of medical care in prisons or mental institutions cruel and unusual punishment?
2. What is "adequate" medical care?
3. Should the same medical standards exist in institutions as in the outside world?
4. Could Kenneth Myers successfully refuse dialysis outside a prison? Could Miriam Winters refuse treatment on the outside? Could the plaintiffs in *Rogers v. Okin*?
5. If noninstitutionalized people know nothing or little about the drugs they take, why would plaintiffs in *Rogers v. Okin* be expected to make competent drug use decisions?
6. What limits exist upon the personal autonomy of confined patients? Why isn't this form of personal privacy absolute?

CHAPTER 6

THE RIGHT TO CHOOSE TREATMENT

INTRODUCTION

FUNDAMENTAL to the concept of informed consent is the idea that the patient should have sufficient information about treatment strategies to be able to choose which treatment he/she desires. Acceptance of this concept, so fundamental to reasonable notions of informed consent and basic to ideas of patient-centered treatment, raises a question: How much freedom should a patient have to choose among alternative treatments? It may be that a patient will be very unwise in his/her choices if total freedom is given the patient. It may also be unreasonable to expect a desperately ill patient to make a rational choice. Such a patient may well grasp for an unproven treatment or unquestioningly accept an extravagant cure claim. These concerns may lead one to restrict the choices available to the patient. At the same time, it must be recognized that new or unusual treatment may be of value in curing an illness or alleviating pain. No physician would likely claim that currently acceptable medical practices include all possible useful treatments for an illness. Thus, to restrict choices of a patient may be to restrict those treatments that are most desirable in caring for the patient.

It may be argued that since it is the patient's body, the patient should be completely free to choose treatments. However, that reasoning presumes that the patient is best able to make such decisions. While it is convenient to believe that this is the case, it must be recognized that society has a role in these choices as well. Society has an interest in its members, and that interest can include the protection of members' lives and health by regulating quackery and unsubstantiated cures.[1]

Practices sometimes found within the collection of therapies known as holistic medicine have presented some of the most complex legal issues questioning the extent to which society can restrict pa-

---

[1]For example, *United States v. Rutherford*, 442 U.S. 544 (1979).

tient choices of treatments. Holistic medicine means that doctors treat patients as an indivisible totality, meeting physical, psychological, social and emotional needs. Treatment of patients is not compartmentalized as is typical of traditional therapies. Nutrition, exercise, and self-regulation techniques form the core of holistic medicine. These therapies embody common sense medical practices and tend to be widely accepted among traditional practitioners. These core therapies also tend to be capable of scientific investigation, and there is scientific support for such techniques. However, the remaining therapies, which include acupuncture, neuromusculature integration, environmental medicine, and spiritual awareness, have very specific applications and are less capable of being subjected to scientific investigation.[2]

Since it is a collection of therapies, a wide spectrum of healthcare practices flourish under the label of holistic medicine. Practitioners of holistic medicine may differ little from traditional practitioners or they may differ dramatically. More radical or faddish treatments include the use of laetrile for cancer, the macrobiotic diet, the laying on of hands, and foot reflexology. The danger of such therapies is not so much that someone will be directly injured by them, but that diagnosis of treatable diseases will be delayed past the point of effective treatment.[3]

Of all nontraditional treatments, laetrile therapy is probably one of the best known and most controversial. Laetrile is an extract of fruit seeds. Its main active ingredient is amygdalin. Proponents of laetrile consider amygdalin to be a vitamin and have labeled it B17. However, it does not demonstrate the chemical action of vitamins. About 6 percent of amygdalin by weight is cyanide. Though the enzyme emulsion needed to release cyanide from amygdalin is not found naturally in the body, it is found in many foods. Thus, cyanide poisoning can be caused by the ingestion of laetrile.[4]

To date, scientific studies have not demonstrated that laetrile has cancer-reducing properties; yet, claims for its curative properties continue. Within the United States, many states have passed stat-

---

[2]Walton, Susan:Holistic medicine (*Science News, 116*:410-412, 1979).
[3]Ibid.
[4]Lerner, Irving J.:Laetrile: A lesson in cancer quackery (*CA-A Cancer Journal for Clinicians, 31*:92-93, 1981).

utes that authorize the use of laetrile.[5] In addition, many Americans travel to other countries such as Mexico for laetrile therapy. The movement to legalize laetrile in the United States has primarily used three pleas for support: (1) cancer patients should have the freedom to choose any therapy they desire; (2) it would be inhumane to withhold hope for cure from a cancer victim; and (3) as a vitamin, laetrile is a dietary choice and not a drug.

The tragedy of young Chad Green, the anonymous child in this chapter's readings, points to the fundamental problem with laetrile. Dependence on laetrile treatment may, in the absence of more traditional treatments, allow cancer to progress until the patient dies.

---

[5]The Food and Drug Administration has recently proposed that Americans returning from foreign countries be allowed to bring back reasonable quantities of unapproved drugs, such as laetrile, for personal use. Keller, Bill: "FDA Seeks to Relax Drug Rule" (*Dallas Times Herald*, October 29, 1982, pp. 1, 20. See also, Ibid., p. 94).

TUMA V. BOARD OF NURSING
OF THE STATE OF IDAHO

(Supreme Court of Idaho, 1979)
No. 12587, April 17, 1979

Is it unprofessional conduct for a nurse to discuss alternative treatments with a patient?

BISTLINE, J.:

"Appellant Tuma challenges an order entered by respondent Board of Nursing (Board) which suspended her registered nurse's license for 6 months, the Board acting on the discussion of a Board-appointed hearing officer who found Tuma guilty of 'unprofessional conduct.'

"During March of 1976, Tuma was employed as a clinical instructor of nursing by the College of Southern Idaho. Her duties included performing nursing services while supervising student nurses at the Twin Falls Clinic and Hospital [Hospital].

"On March 3, 1976, Grace Wahlstrom, a hospital patient, for brevity hereinafter referred to as patient, was informed by her attending physician that she was dying of myelogenous leukemia, that it was malignant, and that her only hope of survival was chemotherapy. She was also told that the drugs involved are life threatening and have undesirable side effects which reduce the body's defense mechanisms, making the patient susceptible to infection and necessitating that the patient be placed in reverse isolation.

"Tuma, aware of the patient's condition and interested in the special needs of dying patients, asked to be assigned to the patient and to administer the prescribed chemotherapy. Tuma discussed the patient's condition and background with her. The patient had fought leukemia for twelve years and attributed her success to her belief in God and to her faithful practice of her religion. They discussed work done by the L.D.S. Hospital in Salt Lake City using chaparral and laetrile, as well as the side effects of the drugs used in the chemotherapy. The patient pleaded with Tuma to return that evening to discuss an alternative treatment using natural products with the patient's family. Tuma consented to the meeting.

"Tuma and a student nurse, Candice Freeman, then commenced the patient's chemotherapy. Freeman testified that Tuma told the patient that discussing these matters 'wasn't exactly ethical.' The patient acknowledged this but still requested Tuma to come back that night. Freeman also testified that Tuma told her to forget what she had heard because it wasn't 'exactly legal.'

"About two hours later, the patient was called by her daughter-in-law, Penny. Penny testified the patient wanted her family to meet Tuma and discuss the alternative treatment. The patient asked Penny not to inform the doctor because this could cause trouble for Tuma. However, Penny called the doctor and informed him of the conversation. He requested that Penny get the name of the nurse, but he did nothing to interfere with the scheduled meeting; nor did he take up the matter with the patient. The doctor ordered the chemotherapy stopped at 8:00 p.m. because of the patient's change of attitude. At 8:00 p.m. that evening, Tuma met with the patient and her family. They discussed the prescribed treatment, its side effects, and the alternatives provided by natural foods and herbs, as well as the fact that the patient would have difficulty getting treatment, particularly blood transfusions, if she left the hospital. Laetrile was discussed as an alternative form of treatment that does not produce the adverse side effects of drugs used in chemotherapy. The patient's son testified that Tuma said her discussion with them was 'somewhat unethical.' After a brief discussion, the parties decided that the patient should remain in the hospital and continue the chemotherapy. The treatment was resumed at 9:15 that evening.

"The patient died two weeks later on March 18, 1976. During the chemotherapy, the patient did experience adverse side effects and was comatose much of the time. There was no contention nor evidence that Tuma's acts in any way contributed to the death of the patient.

* * *

"A hearing was held and...[t]he hearing officer concluded that Tuma 'had violated Idaho Code Section 54-1422 (a) (7), by interfering with the physician-patient relationship and thereby constituting unprofessional conduct....'

"The primary issue on this appeal, and the resolution of which we find to be dispositive, is whether the due process rights of Tuma are satisfied by a statute which authorized the suspension of her professional license to practice nursing on the grounds of 'unprofessional conduct' in the absence of statutes or regulations specifically defining 'unprofessional conduct,' as applied to the conduct which was here held to be unprofessional.

"The right to practice one's profession is a valuable property right. A state cannot exclude a person from the practice of his profession without having provided the safeguards of due process....

* * *

"With respect to Tuma, however, there appears to be no contention whatever that she is unfit to nurse, but rather that she should be punished for the act of talking to the patient about procedures alternative to those which the patient was receiving....

"We find nothing in the statutory definition of 'unprofessional conduct' which can be said to have adequately warned Tuma of the possibility that her license would be suspended if she engaged in conversations with a patient regarding alternative procedures. Hence, it must be held that the statute, unaided by board rules and regulations, does not prohibit the conduct with which she was charged.

* * *

"...As to the charge here leveled against Tuma, that interference with the doctor-patient relationship constitutes unprofessional conduct, again there are no guidelines — nothing which would provide her with sufficient forewarning as to the possibility of license suspension or revocation. We cannot here see how the hearing officer with a legally founded background could properly conclude that Tuma was guilty of unprofessional conduct.

"Nor are we persuaded by the Board's argument that Tuma's guilt could be sufficiently predicated on her own statement that her discussions weren't exactly ethical or legal. Given no written guidelines as to what conduct might possibly result in a suspension of her license for unprofessionalism, Tuma very well may have surmised that she was on thin ice with the particular doctor, or the medical profession in general, in suggesting to a patient alternate procedures for the treatment of cancer. But she could not know, having not even been forewarned against so doing....

* * *

"Shepard, C.J., McFadden, Donaldson, and Bakes, J.J., concur."

CUSTODY OF A MINOR

(Supreme Judicial Court of Massachusetts, 1978)
379 N.E. 2d 1053

May a child be temporarily removed from its parents if they refuse chemotherapy for the child?

HENNESSEY, CHIEF JUSTICE:

* * *

"The facts are as follows: on the evening of August 30, 1977, the child, then twenty months old, awoke with a temperature of 106 degrees. The parents, who were living in Hastings, Nebraska at the time, immediately brought the child to their family physician. Suspecting that the child had leukemia, the physician referred the family to Omaha University Medical Center. On September 1, 1977, physicians at the medical center diagnosed the child's illness as acute lymphocytic leukemia.

"In order to understand the implications of this diagnosis for the child, a more general discussion of the disease and its treatment, as excerpted from the record before us, is helpful. Acute lymphocytic leukemia is a disease of the blood characterized by the appearance in the lymph tissue of excessive numbers of white cells and abnormal cells. The disease is attended by such symptoms as enlargement of the lymph glands, internal bleeding, anemia, and a high susceptibility to infection. Left untreated, the disease is fatal....

"According to uncontroverted medical evidence in this record, the only known medically effective treatment for acute lymphocytic leukemia is chemotherapy, an aggressive three-year treatment program administered in three distinct phases. The first phase is of four week's duration and focuses on killing leukemia cells in the body. In this phase, different anti-leukemia drugs are administered in combination: first, so that the leukemia cells may be attacked at different points in the cell division cycle, and, second, so that the leukemia cells do not develop a resistance to any one drug. The patient in this phase receives two different types of anti-leukemia drugs, one in the form of weekly injections, and another in the form of daily oral dosages.

"The second phase of chemotherapy treatment is six week's long. In this phase, new anti-leukemia drugs are introduced: During the first ten days, a drug called L-Asparaginise is administered intravenously each day; on the eleventh day, and for each successive day during the three-year treatment, a drug called 6-Mercaptopurine is taken orally.

"This second phase of chemotherapy also focuses on attacking leukemia cells which may have migrated into the spinal fluid and which, therefore, may be outside the reach of anti-leukemia drugs which are administered intravenously or by injection. In some treatment programs, cranial radiation is used to attack leukemia cells that may have invaded the central nervous system. In other treatment plans, a drug called Methotrexate® is injected directly into the spinal fluid each week. Thereafter, the drug is taken weekly in pill form until the conclusion of the three-year treatment.

"The third phase of chemotherapy is a maintenance period, which continues until the three years have elapsed. Once during each month of this phase, the patient visits the hospital and receives another combination of anti-leukemia drugs, one in the form of an intravenous injection, and one in the form of an oral dosage taken each day for one week.

"According to the experience of the medical experts in this case, the effect of this type of treatment on the long-term survival of leukemic children has been gratifying. After one year of treatment, 90 percent of the children are found to be disease free. In the second year of treatment, 70 percent are in a state of remission. At the end of the third year, 65 percent are still in remission. In the fourth year, the survival-rate curve flattens to show a steady survival pattern of approximately 50 percent.

"Two other factors are relevant. First, it has been shown that survival rates vary according to the type of leukemia cells found in the child. Because in this case the child is affected with a 'null-cell' type of leukemia, his chances of survival with chemotherapy are slightly higher than 50 percent. Second, because the child falls within an age group which has a higher probability of potential cure and long-term survival, the chances for successful treatment in his case are stronger.

"The child was admitted to a hospital in Omaha on September 1, 1977 and began a program of intensive chemotherapy which anticipated the use of anti-leukemia drugs and cranial radiation. By September 30, 1977, a bone marrow test indicated that the leukemia was in a state of remission.

"In part, because of an aversion to the use of cranial radiation in the child's treatment program, the parents determined in late September that their child's well-being would be best served if the family returned to the father's hometown of Scituate, Massachusetts. The parents made this move on October 8, 1977.

"On October 13, 1977, the family consulted the petitioner, Doctor John T. Truman, Chief of Pediatric Hematology Unit of MGH. After the physician both advised the family that cranial radiation would not be necessary and discussed the chances for cure with chemotherapy, the parents placed the child in Doctor Truman's care. During this visit, Doctor Truman acceded to the parents' request to administer chemotherapy in conjunction with a diet of distilled water, vegetarian foods, and high dosages of vitamins. He explained, however, that while such a diet could be used in addition to chemotherapy, it would have absolutely no value when used alone in the treatment of leukemia.

"The child's treatment at the hospital included injections of a drug called Vincristine® and spinal injections of Methotrexate. Additionally, the parents were instructed to administer a daily 6-Mercaptopurine tablet. During this phase of treatment, bone marrow tests indicated that the child's leukemia was in complete remission. By the second week of November, the child had finished the more vigorous phases of the chemotherapy and the treatment had entered the long-term maintenance phase.

"As a result of the treatment, the child did develop certain side effects, such as stomach cramps and constipation, but these discomforts were alleviated by adjusting the dosages of medication. Additionally, the parents testified to certain short-term behavioral changes in the child, but, in the opinion of the judge, there was no evidence linking these changes to the chemotherapy.

"On November 7, 1977, during one of the child's regular monthly visits to MGH the parents directed Doctor Truman not to administer the scheduled Vincristine injection. Doctor Truman reluctantly agreed and suggested the use of another drug which would involve no injections. A discussion followed, during which the parents asked Doctor Truman what would happen if chemotherapy were terminated. Doctor Truman informed the parents that the chance of relapse in these circumstances was 100 percent.

"By November 10, 1977, the parents stopped giving the child his daily 6-Mercaptopurine tablet. Neither Doctor Truman nor any of the other medical personnel at MGH were informed of this decision. Monthly visits to the hospital continued as scheduled, however.

"During the January hospital visit, Doctor Truman noted changes in the child's condition which suggested that he might not be receiving enough medication. Doctor Truman asked the mother if there had been any difficulty in administering the 6-Mercaptopurine pills. The mother replied that there had been no difficulties, and told Doctor Truman that she needed a new prescription for the medication.

"On February 17, 1978, the parents again brought the child to MGH. The child was pale, was running a temperature, and had developed a cold. Doctor Truman observed that the child's liver was enlarged and that he had developed small hemorrhages under his arm. A blood study revealed the presence of 4 percent leukemia cells. The disease had recurred. After a series of conversations between the parents and Doctor Truman, the mother admitted that they had stopped the child's medication more than three months before.

"During the following four days, Doctor Truman repeatedly telephoned the parents attempting to persuade them to resume the child's treatment. Doctor Truman told them that the chance of cure, while diminished by their cutoff of therapy, still existed, and that their refusal to resume therapy placed a legal responsibility on him as the child's physician. Nevertheless, the parents declined to treat the child.

"On February 22, 1978, the child was brought to MGH pursuant to an order of temporary guardianship issued by the Probate Court. Chemotherapy was resumed, and, as a result, the child's leukemia was again brought into remission. At present, the child continues his treatment program by order of the Superior Court.

***

"...[T]he question whether, and in what circumstances, a State may order medical treatment for a child over parental objections is one of first impression in this Commonwealth. As one commentator points out, the issue places three sets of interests in competion: (1) the 'natural rights' of parents; (2) the responsibilities of the State; and (3) the personal needs of the child. Courts which have considered the question, after balancing these three interests, uniformly have decided that State intervention is appropriate where the medical treatment sought is necessary to save the child's life.

"We conclude that such a decision was also warranted here. First, in determining that intervention was necessary in this case, the judge below gave due weight to the constitutional rights asserted by the parents. Second, the basis of the judge's order, a finding that the parents were unwilling to provide their child with the type of care necessary for his physical well-being, was supported by the evidence. Third, the decision below was consistent with both the best interests of the child and the applicable interests of the State.

"It is well-settled that parents are the 'natural guardians of their children...[with] the legal as well as moral obligation to support... educate and care for the children's development and well-being.... Indeed, these natural rights of parents have been recognized as encompassing an entire 'private realm of family life which must be afforded protection from unwarranted State interference....'

***

"It is also well established, however, that the parental rights described above do not clothe parents with life and death authority over their children.... Thus we have stated that where a child's well-being is placed in issue, 'it is not the rights of parents that are chiefly to be considered. The first and paramount duty is to consult the welfare of the child...'. On a proper showing that parental conduct threatens a child's well-being, the interests of the State and of the individual child may mandate intervention.... [A] child may be taken from the custody of his parents on a showing that 'said child is without necessary and proper physical...care' and that the parents 'are unwilling...to provide such care.' In deciding that such a showing was made here, the judge below essentially found four basic facts: (1) that acute lymphocytic leukemia in children is fatal if untreated; (2) that chemotherapy is the only available medical treatment offering a hope for cure; (3) that the risks of the treatment are minimal when compared to the consequences of allowing the disease to go untreated; and (4) that the parents are unwilling to continue the child's chemotherapy, regardless of the consequences....

* * *

"When considering the question of the child's individual well-being, the judge below applied the doctrine of substituted judgment. By virtue of this doctrine, a court acting on behalf of an incompetent person must first attempt to 'don the mental mantle' of that person, so as to act on 'the same motives and considerations as would have moved [the individual]....'

* * *

"We think that the evidence clearly supported the judge's finding that chemotherapy treatment was in the child's best interest. The judge found several factors weighing in favor of chemotherapy. First, the judge determined that chemotherapy offered the child not only an opportunity for a longer life, but also a 'substantial' chance for cure. Second, the judge considered the child's age, noting that chemotherapy is most effective in the treatment of leukemia in young children, ages one to nine. Third, the judge found that the adverse effects of chemotherapy were minimal. The treatment bore no chance of leaving the child physically incapacitated in any way. Aside from the relatively mild pain associated with constipation and injections, the child suffered no significant side effects from chemotherapy. Indeed, the judge found, after observing the child, that 'but for his underlying condition he appeared to be in perfectly good health, his gait was normal, and his temperament was that of a happy two-year-old.' With treatment, the judge found, the child will be able to attend school, to play, and to engage in the activities of children of his age. Without treatment, the judge found, the child will certainly die.

"The judge identified only two factors weighing against chemotherapy: (1) the possibility of more serious side effects in the future, and (2) the child's inability to understand the significance of the treatment. The judge concluded, however, that neither factor was substantial enough to outweigh chemotherapy. First, according to the evidence, the physical side effects of chemotherapy were found to be controlled and reversible. Second, where the treatment involved was lifesaving in nature, the judge found that the child's inability to understand the temporary pain of chemotherapy could not overcome his long-term interest in leading a normal, healthy life.

"The judge below properly identified three State interests supporting his decision to order medical treatment over parental objections. First, the State has a long-standing interest in protecting the welfare of children living within its borders....

"Second, the State has an interest in the preservation of life. In stressing the importance of this interest, we recognized...that there is a 'substantial distinction in the State's insistence that human life be saved where the affliction is curable,...[and] the State interest where...the issue is not whether, but when, for how long, and at what cost to the individual that life may be briefly extended.' Here, the judge found that the medically indicated treatment program offers the child his only real chance of survival. Consequently, the State interest in the preservation of life applies with full force.

"Third, the State has an interest in protecting the ethical integrity of the medical profession, and in allowing hospitals the full opportunity to care for people under their control....

***

"Judgment affirmed."*

ANDREWS V. BALLARD

(U.S. District Court, 1980)
498 F. Supp. 1038

Is there a fundamental right to obtain acupuncture treatments? If so, may the state limit the practice of acupuncture to licensed physicians?

McDONALD, DISTRICT JUDGE:

***

"Before proceeding to the merits of this action, it may prove useful to review the theory and practice of acupuncture. Acupuncture,

---

*Editor's note: The child was taken by the parents from Massachusetts and received non-traditional treatments for his cancer. The child died.

one branch of traditional Chinese medicine, has been practiced for 2,000 to 5,000 years. It consists of the insertion and manipulation of very fine needles at specific points on or near the surface of the skin. The needles, solid in construction, are usually one to three inches in length, although needles ranging from one-third of an inch to eight inches may be used. They are generally made of stainless steel, although other metals are often employed, and are sterilized before insertion. They may be used to affect the perception of pain (acupuncture analgesia) or to treat certain diseases or dysfunctions (acupuncture therapy).

"The traditional Chinese explanation of how acupuncture works relies heavily on concepts unfamiliar to the Western scientific community. According to traditional Chinese theory, the basic energy or force of life, which flows through all living things, is called 'Ch'i.' when this force flows through the human body, it travels along twelve primary and two secondary channels or meridians. It is along these channels that the acupuncture points lie. Ch'i, traditional Chinese theory teaches, has two aspects to it: Yin, the negative aspect, and Yang, the positive aspect. The twelve primary channels through which Ch'i flows are divided accordingly into six Yin and six Yang channels and paired. For each Yin channel, there is a Yang channel.

"Despite the reference to them as 'negative' and 'positive,' as Yin and Yang are two aspects of the same force, one is no more desirable than the other. In fact, it is a basic tenet of traditional Chinese theory that Yin and Yang must be in balance for Ch'i to flow freely and for all living things, therefore, to function properly. Thus, the theory teaches that it is when Yin and Yang are out of balance that the body is susceptible to pain and illness. Acupuncture treatment is designed to correct this imbalance. The skilled acupuncturist, by placing and manipulating the needles in the proper points, bring Yin and Yang back into balance. This allows Ch'i to flow freely and the body's natural defenses to combat disease and pain.

"Western doctors have advanced a variety of alternative theories as to how acupuncture works.... None of them, however, adequately explain all of acupuncture's manifestations.... [T]he explanation most widely accepted by the 'Western medical community is that acupuncture triggers the production by the pituitary gland of the body's own natural pain-killing substances, endorphins and encephalins, through so-called morphine receptors in the midbrain. But even the endorphin system, although possibly explaining many of the mechanisms of acupuncture, does not account for the specificity of acupuncture since a neurophymoral response might be expected to produce a generalized effect....' Whatever the best explanation is for how acupuncture works, one thing is clear: it does work. All of the evidence put before this Court indicates that, when administered by a skilled practitioner for certain types of pain and dysfunction, acupuncture is both safe and effective.

"...The plaintiffs contend that they have a constitutional right, encompassed by the right of privacy, to decide to obtain or reject medical treatment. That right, they say, protects their decision to obtain acupuncture treatment.

" 'The Constitution,' of course, 'does not explicitly mention any right of privacy. In a line of decisions, however,...the...Court has recognized that a right of personal privacy, or a guarantee of certain zones of privacy,...does exist....' That right is 'one aspect of the "liberty" protected by the Due Process Clause of the Fourteenth Amendment....' As 'an expression of the sanctity of individual free choice and self-determination as fundamental constituents of life,...' it encompasses those interests 'that can be deemed "fundamental" or "implicit" in the concept of ordered liberty....' One such interest is 'the interest in independence in making certain kinds of important decisions....'

***

"...To the extent that the Court has succeeded in that endeavor, it has done so by establishing that the decisions which will be recognized as among those 'that an individual may make without unjustified government interference,...' must meet two criteria. First, they must be 'personal decisions....' They must primarily involve one's self or one's family. Second, they must be 'important decisions....' They must profoundly affect one's development or one's life....

"The decision to obtain or reject medical treatment, no less than the decision to continue or terminate pregnancy, meets both criteria. First, although decisions 'relating to marriage, procreation, contraception, family relationships, and child rearing and education...' often involve and affect other individuals as directly as they do one's self, decisions relating to medical treatment do not. They are, to an extraordinary degree, intrinsically personal. It is the individual making the decision, and no one else, who lives with the pain and disease. It is the individual making the decision, and no one else, who must undergo or forego the treatment. And it is the individual making the decision, and no one else, who, if he or she survives, must live with the results of that decision. One's health is a uniquely personal possession. The decision of how to treat that possession is of a no less personal nature.

"Second, it is impossible to discuss the decision to obtain or reject medical treatment without realizing its importance. The decision can either produce or eliminate physical, psychological, and emotional ruin. It can destroy one's economic stability. It is, for some, the difference between a life of pain and a life of pleasure. It is, for others, the difference between life and death.

"The particular treatment decision involved in the present case, the decision to obtain acupuncture, is of equally substantial import. To begin with, many individuals, including plaintiff John Walker, seek acupuncture only after Western medical techniques have failed them. Doctor Yee-Jung Lok, a Doctor of Traditional Chinese Medicine and master Acupuncturist who presently practices in Nevada and is Chairman of the Advisory Committee to that state's Board of Oriental Medicine, testified that over 90 percent of his patients have previously been treated without success by Western doctors. For these individuals, acupuncture constitutes a last hope. Denied the right to choose acupuncture, they are condemned either to endure without hope the misery that is theirs or to continue to expand their energies and resources on treatment that brings them no relief. The choice is no less important for those who would choose acupuncture over Western medical techniques. The alternative Western treatment, whether drugs or surgery, may involve a serious risk of side effects or injury. For example, a person suffering from severe lower back pain may, denied the choice of acupuncture, be forced to undergo a spinal fusion and risk becoming a virtual invalid for life. Having heard the testimony of plaintiff John Walker, whose suffering and pain brought him to his 'wit's end,' and having seen the videotaped records of five patients of Doctor Yee-Jung Lok, Plaintiffs' Exhibit 1, this Court can only conclude that the decision to obtain acupuncture is one 'fundamentally affecting a person....' One's health is perhaps one's most valuable asset. The importance of decisions affecting it cannot be overstated.

"Thus, the decision to obtain or reject medical treatment, presented in the instant case as the decision to obtain acupuncture treatment, is both personal and important enough to be encompassed by the right of privacy. This should come as no surprise....

* * *

"The fact that the articles and rules in question effectively deprive the plaintiffs of their right to decide to obtain acupuncture treatment does not necessarily, as has been discussed, render them constitutionally infirm. The right of privacy is not absolute.... It may be overcome if the articles and rules being challenged are both motivated by a 'compelling state interest' and 'narrowly drawn to express only' that interest.... In the present case, the plaintiffs concede that the former requirement is met.... [T]he State's interest in preserving and protecting the health of the [patient] may be a 'compelling' one. The question here is whether the State's regulations meet the latter requirement. To do so, they must be 'necessary,...' to the protection of the patient's health.... [T]he challenged rules, it is important to note, are presumably based upon a finding that '[a]cupuncture is an experimental procedure, the safety [and effectiveness] of which [have] not been established....' There are a number of problems with this finding. To begin with, it appears to have been based on no evidence. Doctor Butler testified that the Board of Medical Examiners neither has members who are experts on the theory or practice of acupuncture nor heard testimony by or received evidence from any such experts. Moreover, acupuncture has been practiced for 2000 to 5000 years. It is no more experimental as a mode of medical treatment than is the Chinese language as a mode of communication. What is experimental is not acupuncture, but Westerners' understanding of it and their ability to utilize it properly. Finally, as has been discussed,...all of the evidence adduced before the Court indicates that acupuncture, when administered by a skilled practitioner for certain types of disease and dysfunctions, is both a safe and effective form of medical treatment....

"The defendants argue that the limitation of the practice of acupuncture to licensed physicians...protects against misdiagnoses. Neither patients nor nonphysicians in general, the defendants contend, are as skilled as physicians in diagnosing injuries and illnesses. Thus, the argument goes, it is entirely possible that an individual suffering from cancer would obtain acupuncture treatment for the related pain and that the cancer would continue to spread, undetected by both the patient and the acupuncturist, until it was too late. By requiring the acupuncturist actually to be a licensed physician, the defendants say, the challenged articles and rules help to prevent this situation from occurring. The licensed physician, being trained to recognize the signs of cancer, is more likely to accurately diagnose the disease and arrange for the patient to be treated properly.

"Whether or not the specific scenario envisioned by the defendants is likely to occur, it is possible that the physician-only limitation serves to prevent misdiagnoses. That limitation is not, however, necessary...to prevent such occurrences. The State merely need require that patients consult physicians prior to obtaining acupuncture treatment. At least one state does precisely that....

"The second way in which the physician-only requirement arguably serves to protect patients is by assuring that the acupuncture is administered properly. An acupuncture needle in unskilled hands can cause serious damage. Physicians, the defendants point out, are sworn to preserve health....

"It is rather surprising that the defendants advance this argument. To begin with, the physicians presently practicing in Texas, as a class, are neither skilled nor trained in the practice of acupuncture.... Moreover, there are individuals — acupuncturists — who do have both training and expertise in acupuncture. They are taught where and where not to place acupuncture needles. They know, in other words, how to perform acupuncture. Depending upon the illness or injury involved, they may alter the location of the needles, the depth of insertion, the angle of insertion, the period of insertion, the degree of stimulation to be applied to the needles, the angle of that stimulation, and the association of the needles to each other. According to Doctor Kroening and Doctor Lok, such individuals are currently trained, among other places, in Asia, England, France, Germany, Italy, Sweden, California, and Massachusetts. The foreign locales in which they legally practice include those already mentioned, Australia, Austria, Canada, Switzerland, and New Zealand. In the United States, research indicates, trained acupuncturists are free to practice independently, upon referral from a licensed physician, or under the supervision of a licensed physician, in Arizona, California, the District of Columbia, Florida, Hawaii, Louisiana, Massachusetts, Montana, Nevada, New York, Oregon, Rhode Island, South Carolina, Tennessee and Washington.

***

"The third way in which the challenged articles and rules theoretically protect the patient's health is by assuring that any complications which may arise during acupuncture treatment will be remedied as quickly as possible....

"The articles and rules are not, however, 'tailored'...to the achievement of that objective. The State has made no effort to determine what type of complications, if any, arise during acupuncture. It has taken no steps to assure that physicians are trained to deal with those types of complications. It has made no determination that other individuals, such as trained acupuncturists, are not equally able to remedy those types of complications. And it has done nothing to prevent such complications from occurring in the first place. There are clearly 'less drastic means'...the State could take to avoid the danger involved here. It could require acupuncturists to make arrangements to have emergency medical treatment readily available, or, if it truly considered the presence of a physician essential, it could enact regulations requiring acupuncturists to assure that their patients have ready access to a physician. The State, however, has not done this....

***

"So long as it does not significantly interfere with...the decision to obtain the treatment, the State of Texas is, of course, free to deal with acupuncture as it chooses. It may accord to acupuncturists, as it does to chiropractors,...full independent professional status. It may allow acupuncturists to practice independently of licensed physicians, but require diagnosis by or referral from such physicians. It may establish appropriate minimum standards of skill and knowledge to be met by those who practice acupuncture. It may even, if it considers such a framework feasible, require acupuncturists to practice under the supervision and control of licensed physicians.... It may choose to regulate acupuncture in some entirely different fashion, or not at all. What it may not do, what it has done in the present case, is to unnecessarily render acupuncture treatment essentially unavailable. That the Constitution prohibits."

* * *

MATTER OF HOFBAUER

(Court of Appeals of New York, 1979)
393 N.E. 2d 1009

May a child be found neglected if he is treated by a physician who advocated diet and laetrile therapy for Hodgkin's disease rather than traditional treatments?

JASEN, JUDGE:

"This appeal involves the issue whether a child suffering from Hodgkin's disease whose parents failed to follow the recommendation of an attending physician to have their child treated by radiation and chemotherapy, but, rather, placed their child under the care of physicians advocating nutritional or metabolic therapy, including injections of laetrile, is a 'neglected child' within the meaning of section 1012 of the Family Court Act. This case does not involve the legality of the use of laetrile *per se* in this State inasmuch as neither party contends that a duly licensed New York physician may not administer laetrile to his or her own patients. Nor is this an action brought against a physician to test the validity of his determination to treat Hodgkin's disease by prescribing metabolic therapy and injections of laetrile. Rather, the issue presented for our determination is whether the parents of a child afflicted with Hodgkin's disease have failed to exercise a minimum degree of care in supplying their child with adequate medical care by entrusting the child's physical well-being to a duly licensed physician who advocates a treatment not widely embraced by the medical community.

"The relevant facts are as follows: In October, 1977, Joseph Hofbauer, then a seven-year-old child, was diagnosed as suffering from Hodgkin's disease, a disease which is almost always fatal if left untreated. The then attending physician, Doctor Arthur Cohn, recommended that Joseph be seen by an oncologist or hematologist for further treatment which would have included radiation treatments and possibly chemotherapy, the conventional modes of treatment. Joseph's parents, however, after making numerous inquiries, rejected Doctor Cohn's advice and elected to take Joseph to Fairfield Medical Clinic in Jamaica where a course of nutritional or metabolic therapy, including injection of laetrile, was initiated.

***

"A reading of this statutory provision makes it clear that the Legislature has imposed upon the parents of a child the non-delegable affirmative duty to provide their child with adequate medical care. What constitutes adequate medical care, however, cannot be judged in a vacuum free from external influences, but, rather, each case must be decided on its own particular facts. In this regard, we deem certain factors significant in determining whether Joseph was afforded adequate medical care.

"...[I]t is important to stress that a parent, in making the sensitive decision as to how the child should be treated, may rely upon the recommendations and competency of the attending physician if he or she is duly licensed to practice medicine in this State, for '[i]f a physician is licensed by the State, he is recognized by the State as capable of exercising acceptable clinical judgment....'

"...[I]n our view, the court's inquiry should be whether the parents, once having sought accredited medical assistance and having been made aware of the seriousness of their child's affliction and the possibility of cure if a certain mode of treatment is undertaken, have provided for their child a treatment which is recommended by their physician and which has not been totally rejected by all responsible medical authority.

***

"...[A]ppellants predicate their charge of neglect upon the basis that Joseph's parents have selected for their child a mode of treatment which is inadequate and ineffective. Both courts below found, however — and we conclude that these findings are supported by the record — that numerous qualified doctors have been consulted by Doctor Schachter and have contributed to the child's care; that the parents have both serious and justifiable concerns about the deleterious effects of radiation treatments and chemotherapy; that there is medical proof that the nutritional treatment being administered

Joseph was controlling his condition and that such treatment is not as toxic as is the conventional treatment; and that conventional treatments will be administered to the child if his condition so warrants. In light of these affirmed findings of fact, we are unable to conclude, as a matter of law, that Joseph's parents have not undertaken reasonable efforts to ensure that acceptable medical treatment is being provided their child."

***

UNITED STATES V. RUTHERFORD

(U.S. Supreme Court, 1979)
442 U.S. 544

The Federal Food, Drug, and Cosmetic Act prohibits interstate distribution of any new drug whose safety and effectiveness has not been substantiated. Terminally ill cancer patients sought to have laetrile exempted from the Act's prohibition of interstate distribution. The District Court and the Court of Appeals held that the exemption should be granted. These rulings were reversed.

JUSTICE MARSHALL:

***

"...He [FDA Commissioner] determined first that no uniform definition of laetrile exists; rather, the term has been used generically for chemical compounds similar to, or consisting at least in part of, amygdalin, a glucoside present in the kernels or seeds of most fruits.... The Commissioner further found that laetrile in its various forms constituted a 'new drug' as defined in §201(p)(1) of the Act because it was not generally recognized among experts as safe and effective for its prescribed use....

"Having determined that laetrile was a new drug, the Commissioner proceeded to consider whether it was exempt from premarketing approval under the 1938 or 1962 grandfather provisions.... First, there was no showing that the drug currently known as laetrile was identical in composition or labeling to any drug distributed before 1938.... Nor could the Commissioner conclude from the evidence submitted that, as of October 9, 1962, laetrile in its present chemical composition was commercially used or sold in the United

States, was generally recognized by experts as safe, and was labeled for the same recommended uses as the currently marketed drug....

* * *

"...[T]he court held that, by denying cancer patients the right to use a nontoxic substance in connection with their personal health, the Commissioner had infringed constitutionally protected privacy interests....

"The Court of Appeals addressed neither the statutory nor the constitutional rulings of the District Court. Rather, the Tenth Circuit held that the 'safety' and 'effectiveness' terms used in the statute have no reasonable application to terminally ill cancer patients.... since those patients, by definition, would 'die of cancer regardless of what may be done,' the court concluded that there were no realistic standards against which to measure the safety and effectiveness of a drug for that class of individuals....

* * *

"...In the instant case, we are persuaded by the legislative history and consistent administrative interpretation of the Act that no implicit exemption for drugs used by the terminally ill is necessary to attain congressional objectives or to avert an unreasonable reading of the terms 'safe' and 'effective'....

* * *

"In the Court of Appeals' view, an implied exemption from the Act was justified because the safety and effectiveness §201(p)(1) could have 'no reasonable application' to terminally ill patients.... We disagree. Under our constitutional framework, federal courts do not sit as councils of revision, empowered to rewrite legislation in accord with their own conceptions of prudent public policy.... Only when a literal construction of a statute yields results so manifestly unreasonable that they could not fairly be attributed to congressional design will an exception to statutory language be judicially implied.... Here, however, we have no license to depart from the plain language of the Act, for Congress could reasonably have intended to shield terminal patients from ineffectual or unsafe drugs.

* * *

"Moreover, there is a special sense in which the relationship between drug effectiveness and safety has meaning in the context of incurable illnesses. An otherwise harmless drug can be dangerous to any patient if it does not produce its purported therapeutic effect.... But if an individual suffering from a potentially fatal disease rejects conventional therapy in favor of a drug with no demonstrable curative properties, the consequences can be irreversible. For this reason, even before the 1962 Amendments incorporated an efficacy standard into new drug application procedures, the FDA considered effectiveness when reviewing the safety of drugs used to treat terminal illness.... The FDA's practice also reflects the recognition, amply supported by expert medical testimony in this case, that with diseases such as cancer it is often impossible to identify a patient as terminally ill except in retrospect. Cancers vary considerably in behavior and in responsiveness to different forms of therapy.... Even critically ill individuals may have unexpected remissions and may respond to conventional treatment.... Thus, as the Commissioner concluded, 'to exempt from the Act drugs with no proved effectiveness in the treatment of cancer would lead to needless deaths and suffering among...patients characterized as 'terminal' who would actually be helped by legitimate therapy....'

"It bears emphasis that although the Court of Appeals' ruling was limited to laetrile, its reasoning cannot be so readily confined. To accept the proposition that the safety and efficacy standards of the Act have no relevance for terminal patients is to deny the Commissioner's authority over all drugs, however toxic or ineffectual, for such individuals. If history is any guide, this new market would not be long overlooked. Since the turn of the century, resourceful entrepreneurs have advertised a wide variety of purportedly simple and painless cures for cancer, including liniments of turpentine, mustard, oil, eggs, and ammonia; peat moss; arrangements of colored floodlamps; pastes made from glycerin and limburger cheese; mineral tablets, and 'Fountain of Youth' mixtures of spices, oil, and suet. In citing these examples, we do not, of course, intend to deprecate the sincerity of laetrile's current proponents, or to imply any opinion on whether that drug may ultimately prove safe and effective for cancer treatment. But this historical experience does suggest why Congress could reasonably have determined to protect the terminally ill, no less than other patients, from the vast range of self-styled panaceas that inventive minds can devise.

"We note finally that construing §201(p)(1) to encompass treatments for terminal diseases do not foreclose all resort to experimental cancer drugs by patients for whom conventional therapy is unavailable. Section 505(i) of the Act...exempts from premarketing approval drugs intended solely for investigative use if they satisfy certain preclinical testing and other criteria....

"The judgment of the Court of Appeals is reversed, and the case is remanded for further proceedings consistent with this opinion. So ordered."

QUESTIONS

1. Why is there an assumption in *U.S. v. Rutherford* (1979) that terminally ill patients will be exploited by unscrupulous cure-all dealers? Could it alternatively be assumed that terminally ill patients will be free to make a choice? If they choose laetrile, is that not part of their liberty to choose?

2. If Joseph Hofbauer's parents treated him with diet and laetrile, without the advice of a physician, would they be guilty of neglect? Why does a physician's involvement legitimize the treatment? Suppose Joseph's disease was not in remission, would the court have decided differently?

3. Does *Andrews v. Ballard* make state regulation of medicine extraordinarily difficult?

4. Why is there a fundamental right to acupuncture, but not laetrile?

5. Is *Hofbauer* similar to *Custody of a Minor*? Why is there a right to choose alternative treatments in *Hofbauer*, but not in *Custody of a Minor*?

6. To what extent should a nurse discuss treatment alternatives with patients and/or their families?

CHAPTER 7

THE RIGHT TO DIE

INTRODUCTION

OTHER than abortion, the right to die has probably received more popular attention than any other legal-medical issue. The right to die essentially accepts the premise that life can be so unsatisfactory that it should not be prolonged. In fact, many religions accept the view that the process of dying should not be unnecessarily prolonged. The Catholic church, for example, teaches that extraordinary measures do not need to be undertaken to prolong the life of the dying. In the Jewish rabbinical tradition, there is not a clear toleration of any withdrawal of treatment. However, a state of *gesisah* is recognized where the ill person has become moribund and where death is imminent. During the state of *gesisah*, one may withdraw the impediments to dying. It is said that the chopping of wood keeps the soul from departing the body. During *gesisah* it would be permissible to keep such sounds from the patient. Generally, it might be said, Protestant theologians would also recognize that dying should not be unnecessarily prolonged, and that there is a point where treatment must stop so that the patient may be allowed to die.[1]

Several courts have attempted to make the concept of withdrawal of medical treatment into a legal right. At times, it would appear that some courts have gone well beyond religious traditions and have authorized a right to die even though death was not clearly imminent or was avoidable. In general, it is possible to divide right-to-die cases into two types. One type is best illustrated by *Matter of Quinlan*.[2] Karen Quinlan was clearly incapable of recovery from her vegetative state. When her father sought to be named her guardian and remove life-support systems, it was with the firm belief that the life-support systems were only unnecessarily prolonging Karen Quinlan's death. Mr. Quinlan had consulted a priest prior to going to court and was following the teaching of the Catholic church. In

---

[1]Veatch, Robert M.:*A Theory of Medical Ethics* (New York, Basic Books, 1981, pp. 27-43).
[2]*Matter of Quinlan*, 355 A. 2d 647 (1976).

allowing life-support systems to be withdrawn, the New Jersey Supreme Court recognized that there was a right to die. That Karen Quinlan did not die when life-support systems were withdrawn should not detract from the belief by Mr. Quinlan and the Court that those systems were keeping her alive unnecessarily and that there was no hope that her condition would improve. Other cases have built on *Quinlan's* recognition of a right to die, although factual differences have existed which have led to some questioning of the breadth of the right to die.

Quinlan raises a significant question about the meaning of "extraordinary measures." It was argued, and a Catholic Bishop among others agreed, that Karen's respirator was an extraordinary measure that was unnecessarily and hopelessly prolonging her life. Yet, Karen continues to receive feedings and antibiotics to ward off infections that would surely kill her. It could be argued that the feedings or the antibiotics are also extraordinary. It is probably impossible to reach complete agreement on what treatments are extraordinary and what are not. Decisions of this sort will likely vary with the times and with the circumstances of each case. However, the flexibility of the term provides opportunities for the exercise of discretion by medical personnel. It also provides enormous opportunities for litigation over the meaning of the term in specific situations.

There is another type of right-to-die case that is quite different from *Quinlan* and its related cases. That case type is probably best illustrated by the *Baby Doe* case.[3] Baby Doe was a Down's syndrome baby who also suffered from a fatal digestive defect. The defect was correctable by surgery which was not considered to be particularly complex or particularly dangerous. Without that surgery, death for Baby Doe was imminent. With that surgery, Baby Doe would have likely lived, although it would have been the life of a Down's syndrome child. Rather than allow the surgery, the parents chose to exercise their right to refuse to grant permission for the surgery. After several days, Baby Doe starved to death.

The justification for allowing people, such as Baby Doe, to die comes from a distinction that is made between active and passive euthanasia. Active euthanasia within a medical setting is probably quite rare. Indeed, if discovered, one who engages in active eu-

---

[3] Regretfully, the Indiana Supreme Court issued no opinion in the case and sealed all records.

thanasia is probably subject to murder charges. Passive euthanasia, on the other hand, is quite common within a medical setting.[4] The difference between the two types is probably best pointed out by an example. If a patient is dying, a physician might administer a lethal injection to put an end to the patient's suffering. That action, however, would be active euthanasia and would subject the physician to criminal charges. On the other hand, it may be that a patient is dying, although drugs may be able to briefly prolong his life and his suffering. A doctor may decide not to administer any medication. By doing nothing, the patient will die and his/her suffering will be reduced. Such failure to act would be passive euthanasia. The difference between the two, many will argue, is that with passive euthanasia, the illness is the cause of the patient's death. The physician is not the cause of death because he/she did nothing to cause death. Instead, the physician merely stood aside and awaited the normal course of the illness. Critics of this view would argue that there is no difference between active and passive because in both cases the consequence is death. A physician, it is argued, is responsible for the patient and is responsible for the patient's death whether that death is the result of the physician's lethal injection or whether the doctor did nothing but stand at the patient's bedside.[5] Cases such as *Baby Doe* require a recognition of a valid distinction between active and passive euthanasia. Without such a distinction, the criminal laws protecting human life would appear to be applicable.

Passive euthanasia is common and, as several of the cases in this chapter point out, it has been legitimized by courts. It can be argued, however, that active euthanasia is far more humane than passive. Note that Baby Doe starved for days before dying. Rather than allowing one to die, such as Baby Doe, by causing days of suffering for the infant, a lethal injection might be more desirable. If death is to be allowed to occur, there may be an obligation to reduce the suffering associated with death. One might argue against both

'Rachels, James: Euthanasia, killing and letting die. In Ladd, John (Ed.):*Ethical Issues Relating to Life and Death* (New York, Oxford, 1979, pp. 146-163); Ladd, John: Positive and negative euthanasia. In Ladd, John (Ed.):*Ethical Issues Relating to Life and Death* (New York, Oxford, 1979, pp. 164-186); Foot, Philippa: Euthanasia. In McMullin (Ed.):*Death and Decision* (Boulder, Westview, 1978, pp. 85-110).
'Ladd, Op cit., pp. 164-166.

points by taking the position that human life is sacred and that medical efforts must be undertaken to prolong all human lives. Advocates of such a position would argue that neither action to bring about death or inaction which would allow death is appropriate. Such a position, however, ignores the suffering that would be prolonged among the dying.[6]

In order to provide some background for understanding what happened in the *Baby Doe* case, it should be noted that Down's syndrome children usually have IQ's that range between 25 and 50. Generally, Down's syndrome children are educable or trainable.[7] They also have a low life expectancy.

Down's syndrome can be diagnosed early in pregnancy by examining fetal cells obtained from amniotic fluid. It is likely that many women choose an early-term abortion rather than give birth to a Down's syndrome baby. Spontaneous abortions of Down's syndrome fetuses are also quite common. As many as 50 percent of first-trimester spontaneous abortions are due to genetic defects. There is a much higher chance of spontaneous abortion during the second half of pregnancy for a Down's fetus compared to a normal fetus.

The *Baby Doe* case has led the federal government to warn hospitals that such cases may violate the law, which forbids discrimination against the handicapped. One clear concern that should be raised by such cases is whether the right to die has become a right to let defective children die.

Though the *Baby Doe* case involved Down's syndrome, one can think of relatively uncommon genetic diseases where both child and parents would be even more burdened. For example, Tay-Sachs disease is a genetic disease characterized by an error in fat metabolism that leads to a fatty accumulation around the cells of the nervous system. It is an incurable disease that at six months leaves a child apathetic and without muscle tone. The disease progresses and the child becomes blind, quadriplegic, and lapses into a vegetative state. The child will likely die by his third birthday after leading a life filled with suffering. Severe forms of spina bifida result in loss of nerve function for children and varying degrees of paralysis, some near to-

---

⁷Ibid., pp. 183-184.

tal paralysis. Without treatment, a severe spina bifida child will probably die from infection. With treatment, a child can live but often with severe paralysis and serious neurological defects.[7] If treatment should be withdrawn from such children, where does one draw the line?

---

[7]For a discussion of defective newborns, including Down's syndrome, Tay-Sachs and spina bifida babies, see Ramsey, Paul:*Ethics at the Edges of Life* (New Haven, Yale, 1978, pp. 189-227).

MATTER OF QUINLAN

(Supreme Court of New Jesey, 1976)
355 A. 2d 647

May the father of a comatose patient with no chance of recovery be named guardian of the patient for the purpose of removing her from life-support systems?

CHIEF JUSTICE HUGHES:

* * *

"On the night of April 15, 1975, for reasons still unclear, Karen Quinlan ceased breathing for at least two 15-minute periods. She received some ineffectual mouth-to-mouth resuscitation from friends. She was taken by ambulance to Newton Memorial Hospital. There she had a temperature of 100 degrees. Her pupils were unreactive and she was unresponsive even to deep pain. The history at the time of her admission to that hospital was essentially incomplete and uninformative.

"Three days later, Doctor Morse examined Karen at the request of the Newton admitting physician, Doctor McGee. He found her comatose with evidence of decortication, a condition relating to derangement of the cortex of the brain causing a physical posture in which the upper extremities are flexed and the lower extremities are extended. She required a respirator to assist her breathing....An electroencephalogram (EEG) measuring electrical rhythm of the brain was performed, and Doctor Morse characterized the result as 'abnormal but it showed some activity and was consistent with her clinical state.' Other significant neurological tests, including a brain scan, an angiogram, and a lumbar puncture were normal in result.... Karen was originally in a sleep-like unresponsive condition but soon developed 'sleep-wake' cycles, apparently a normal improvement for comatose patients occurring within three to four weeks. In the awake cycle she blinks, cries out and does things of that sort but is still totally unaware of anyone or anything around her.

"Doctor Morse and other expert physicians who examined her characterized Karen as being in a 'chronic persistent vegetative state.' Doctor Fred Plum, one of such expert witnesses, defined this as a 'subject who remains with the capacity to maintain the vegetative parts of neurological function but who no longer has any cognitive function.'

"Doctor Morse, as well as the several other medical and neurological experts who testified in this case, believed with certainty that Karen Quinlan is not 'brain dead....'

* * *

"The experts believe that Karen cannot now survive without the assistance of the respirator; that exactly how long she would live without it is unknown; that the strong likelihood is that death would follow soon after its removal, and that removal would also risk further brain damage and would curtail the assistance the respirator presently provides in warding off infection.

* * *

"It is the issue of the constitutional right of privacy that has given us most concern, in the exceptional circumstances of this case. Here a loving parent, *qua* parent and raising the rights of his incompetent and profoundly damaged daughter, probably irreversibly doomed to no more than a biologically vegetative remnant of life, is before the court. He seeks authorization to abandon specialized technological procedures which can only maintain for a time a body having no potential for resumption or continuance of other than a 'vegetative' existence.

"We have no doubt, in these unhappy circumstances, that if Karen were herself miraculously lucid for an interval (not altering the existing prognosis of the condition to which she would soon return) and perceptive of her irreversible condition, she could effectively decide upon discontinuance of the life-support apparatus, even if it meant the prospect of natural death....

"[N]o external compelling interest of the State could compel Karen to endure the unendurable, only to vegetate a few measurable months with no realistic possibility of returning to any semblance of cognitive or sapient life. We perceive no thread of logic distinguishing between such a choice on Karen's part and a similar choice which...could be made by a competent patient terminally ill, riddled by cancer and suffering great pain; such a patient would not be resuscitated or put on a respirator...and *a fortiori* would not be kept against his will on a respirator.

* * *

"The claimed interests of the State in this case are essentially the preservation and sanctity of human life and defense of the right of the physician to administer medical treatment according to his best judgment. In this case the doctors say that removing Karen from the respirator will conflict with their professional judgment.... The nature of Karen's care and the realistic chance of her recovery are quite unlike those of the patient discussed in many of the cases where treatments were ordered. In many of those cases the medical procedure required (usually a transfusion) constituted a minimal bodily invasion and the chances of recovery and return to functioning life were very good. We think that the State's interest *contra* weakens and the individual's right to privacy grows as the degree of bodily invasion increases and the prognosis dims. Ultimately there comes a point at which the individual's rights overcome the State interest....

"Our affirmation of Karen's independent right of choice, however, would ordinarily be based upon her competency to assert it. The sad truth, however, is that she is grossly incompetent and we cannot discern her supposed choice based on the testimony of her previous conversations with friends, where such testimony is without sufficient probative weight.... Nevertheless we have concluded that Karen's right of privacy may be asserted on her behalf by her guardian under the peculiar circumstances here present.

"If a putative decision by Karen to permit this non-cognitive, vegetative existence to terminate by natural forces is regarded as a valuable incident of her right of privacy, as we believe it to be, then it should not be discarded solely on the basis that her condition prevents her conscious exercise of the choice. The only practical way to prevent destruction of the right is to permit the guardian and family of Karen to render their best judgment, subject to the qualifications hereinafter stated, as to whether she would exercise it in these circumstances. If their conclusion is in the affirmative, this decision should be accepted by a society the overwhelming majority of whose members would, we think, in similar circumstances, exercise such a choice in the same way for themselves or for those closest to them. It is for this reason that we determine that Karen's right of privacy may be asserted in her behalf, in this respect, by her guardian and family under the particular circumstances presented by this record.

***

"...The physicians in charge of the case...declined to withdraw the respirator. That decision was consistent with...the then existing medical standards and practices.

***

"However, in relation to the matter of the declaratory relief sought by plaintiff as representative of Karen's interest, we are required to reevaluate the applicability of the medical standards projected in the court below. The question is whether there is such internal consistency and rationality in the application of such standards as should warrant their constituting an inelectable bar to the effectuation of substantive relief for plaintiff at the hands of the court. We have concluded not.

***

"The modern proliferation of substantial malpractice litigation and the less frequent but even more unnerving possibility of criminal sanctions would seem, to have bearing on the practice and standards as they exist. The possible liability, it was testified here, had no part in the decision of the treating physicians.... But we cannot believe that the stated factor has not had a strong influence on the standards, as the literature on the subject plainly reveals.... Moreover our attention is drawn not so much to the recognition by Doctors Morse and Javed of the extant practice and standards but to the widening ambiguity of those standards themselves in their application to the medical problems we are discussing.

***

"We glean from the record here that physicians distinguish between curing the ill and comforting and easing the dying: that they refuse to treat the curable as if they were dying or ought to die, and that they have sometimes refused to treat the hopeless and dying as if they were curable. In this sense, as we were reminded by the testimony of Doctors Korein and Diamond, many of them have refused to inflict an undesired prolongation of the process of dying on a patient in irreversible condition when it is clear that such 'therapy' offers neither human nor humane benefit. We think these attitudes represent a balanced implementation of a profoundly realistic perspective on the meaning of life and death and that they respect the whole Judeo-Christian tradition of regard for human life. No less would they seem consistent with the moral matrix of medicine, 'to heal,' very much in the sense of the endless mission of the law, 'to do justice.'

"Yet this balance, we feel, is particularly difficult to perceive and apply in the context of the development by advanced technology of sophisticated and artificial life-sustaining devices. For those possibly curable, such devices are of great value, and, as ordinary medical procedures, are essential. Consequently, as pointed out by Doctor Diamond, they are necessary because of the ethic of medical practice. But in light of the situation in the present case...one would have to think that the use of the same respirator or life support would be considered 'ordinary' in the context of the possibly curable patient but 'extraordinary' in the context of the forces sustaining by cardio-respiratory processes of an irreversibly doomed patient. And this dilemma is sharpened in the face of the malpractice and criminal action threat which we have mentioned.

"We would hesitate, in this imperfect world, to propose as to physicians that type of immunity which from the early common law has surrounded judges and grand jurors...so that they might without fear of personal retaliation perform their judicial duties with independent objectivity....

"Nevertheless, there must be a way to free physicians, in the pursuit of their healing vocation, from possible contamination by self-interest or self-protection concerns which would inhibit their independent medical judgments for the well-being of their dying patients....

***

"The most appealing factor in the technique suggested by Doctor Teel (an Ethics Committe which would serve as a regular forum for discussion of the ethical problems of individual cases) seems to us to be the diffusion of professional responsibility for decision, comparable in a way to the value of multi-judge courts in finally resolving on appeal difficult questions of law. Moreover, such a system would be protective to the hospital as well as the doctor in screening out, so to speak, a case which might be contaminated by less than worthy motivations of family or physician. In the real world and in relationship to the momentous decision contemplated, the value of additional views and diverse knowledge is apparent.

"We consider that a practice of applying to a court to confirm such decisions would generally be inappropriate, not only because that would be a gratuitous encroachment upon the medical profession's field of competence, but because it would be impossibly cumbersome. Such a requirement is distinguishable from the judicial overview traditionally required in other matters such as the adjudication and commitment of mental incompetents. This is not to say that in the case of an otherwise justiciable controversy access to the courts would be foreclosed; we speak rather of a general practice and procedure.

"And although the deliberations and decisions which we describe would be professional in nature they should obviously include at some stage the feelings of the family of an incompetent relative....

* * *

"Having concluded that there is a right of privacy that might permit termination of treatment in the circumstances of this case, we turn to consider the relationship of the exercise of that right to the criminal law. We are aware that such termination of treatment would accelerate Karen's death.... We conclude that there would be no criminal homicide in the circumstances of this case. We believe, first, that the ensuing death would not be homicide but rather expiration from existing natural causes. Secondly, even if it were to be regarded as homicide, it would not be unlawful.

* * *

"...We do not question the State's power to punish the taking of human life, but that power does not encompass individuals terminating medical treatment pursuant to their right of privacy.... The constitutional protection extends to third parties whose action is necessary to effectuate the exercise of that right where the individuals themselves would not be subject to prosecution or the third parties are charged as accessories to an act which could not be a crime....

* * *

"...[W]e herewith declare the following affirmative relief on behalf of the plaintiff. Upon the concurrence of the guardian and family of Karen, should the responsible attending physicians conclude that there is no reasonable possibility of Karen's ever emerging from her present comatose condition to a cognitive, sapient state and that the life-support apparatus not being administered to Karen should be discontinued, they shall consult with the hospital 'Ethics Committee' or like body of the institution in which Karen is then hospitalized. If that consultative body agrees that there is no reasonable possibility of Karen's ever emerging from her present comatose condition to a cognitive sapient state, the present life-support system may be withdrawn and said action shall be without any civil or criminal liability therefore on the part of any participant, whether guardian, physician, hospital or others...."*

SUPERINTENDENT OF BELCHERTOWN V. SAIKEWICZ

(Supreme Judicial Court of Massachusetts, 1977)
370 N.E. 2d 417

May a severely retarded adult male be allowed to die rather than undergo cancer therapy?

JUSTICE LIACOS:

* * *

"...Joseph Saikewicz, at the time the matter arose, was sixty-seven years old, with an IQ of ten and a mental age of approximately two years and eight months. He was profoundly mentally retarded. The record discloses that, apart from his leukemic condition, Saikewicz enjoyed generally good heatlh. He was physically strong and well built, nutritionally nourished, and ambulatory. He was not, however, able to communicate verbally — resorting to gestures and grunts to make his wishes known to others and responding only to gestures or physical contacts. In the course of treatment for

---

*Editors' note: Karen Quinlan was removed from life-support systems. She continues to live. She currently receives care in a nursing home since she remains in a comatose state. No effort has been made to deny Karen nourishment or the antibiotics necessary to combat the ever-present danger of serious and possibly fatal infections.

various medical conditions arising during Saikewicz's residency at the school, he had been unable to respond intelligibly to inquiries such as whether he was experiencing pain. It was the opinion of a consulting psychologist, not contested by the other experts relied on by the judge below, that Saikewicz was not aware of dangers and was disoriented outside of his immediate environment. As a result of his condition, Saikewicz had lived in State institutions since 1923 and had resided at the Belchertown State School since 1928. Two of his sisters, the only members of his family who could be located, were notified of his condition and of the hearing, but they preferred not to attend or otherwise become involved.

"On April 19, 1976, Saikewicz was diagnosed as suffering from acute myeloblastic monocytic leukemia. Leukemia is a disease of the blood. It arises when organs of the body produce an excessive number of white blood cells as well as other abnormal cellular structures, in particular undeveloped and immature white cells. Along with these symptoms in the composition of the blood the disease is accompanied by enlargement of the organs which produce the cells (e.g. the spleen, lymph glands, and bone marrow). The disease tends to cause internal bleeding and weakness, and, in the acute form, severe anemia and high susceptibility to infection.... The particular form of the disease present in this case...is invariably fatal.

"Chemotherapy, as was testified to at the hearing in the Probate Court, involves the administration of drugs over several weeks, the purpose of which is to kill the leukemia cells. This treatment unfortunately affects normal cells as well. One expert testified that the end result, in effect, is to destroy the living vitality of the bone marrow. Because of this effect, the patient becomes very anemic and may bleed or suffer infections — a condition which requires a number of blood transfusions. In this sense, the patient immediately becomes much 'sicker' with the commencement of chemotherapy, and there is a possibility that infections during the initial period of severe anemia will prove fatal. Moreover, while most patients survive chemotherapy, remission of the leukemia is achieved in only 30 to 50 percent of the cases. Remission is meant here as a temporary return to normal as measured by clinical and laboratory means. If remission does occur, it typically lasts for between two and thirteen months, although longer periods of remission are possible. Estimates of

the effectiveness of chemotherapy are complicated in cases such as the one presented here, in which the patient's age becomes a factor. According to the medical testimony before the court below, persons over age sixty have more difficulty tolerating chemotherapy and the treatment is likely to be less successful than in younger patients.*
This prognosis may be compared with the doctor's estimates that, left untreated, a patient in Saikewicz's condition would live for a matter of weeks or, perhaps, several months. According to the testimony, a decision to allow the disease to run its natural course would not result in pain for the patient, and death would probably come without discomfort.

"An important facet of the chemotherapy process, to which the judge below directed careful attention, is the problem of serious adverse side effects caused by the treating drugs. Among these side effects are severe nausea, bladder irritation, numbness and tingling of the extremities, and loss of hair. The bladder irritation can be avoided, however, if the patient drinks fluids, and the nausea can be treated by drugs. It was the opinion of the guardian *ad litem*, as well as the doctors who testified before the probate judge, that most people elect to suffer the side effects of chemotherapy rather than to allow their leukemia to run its natural course.

"Drawing on the evidence before him including the testimony of the medical experts, and the report of the guardian *ad litem*, the probate judge issued detailed findings with regard to the costs and benefits of allowing Saikewicz to undergo chemotherapy....

* * *

"...[T]he judge concluded that the following considerations weighed against administering chemotherapy to Saikewicz: '(1) his age, (2) his inability to cooperate with the treatment, (3) probable adverse side effects of treatment, (4) low chance of producing remission, (5) the certainty that treatment will cause immediate suffering, and (6) the quality of life possible for him even if the treatment does bring about remission.'

"The following considerations were determined to weigh in favor of chemotherapy: '(1) the chance that his life may be lengthened

---

*On appeal, the petitioners have collected in their brief a number of recent empirical studies which cast doubt on the view that patients over sixty are less successfully treated by chemotherapy....

thereby, and (2) the fact that most people in his situation when given a chance to do so elect to take the gamble of treatment.'

"Concluding that, in this case, the negative factors of treatment exceeded the benefits, the probate judge ordered on May 13, 1976, that no treatment be administered to Saikewicz for his condition of acute myeloblastic monocytic leukemia except by further order of the court. The judge further ordered that all reasonable and necessary supportive measures be taken, medical or otherwise, to safeguard the well-being of Saikewicz in all other respects and to reduce as far as possible any suffering or discomfort which he might experience.

* * *

"The current state of medical ethics in this area is expressd by one commentator who states that: 'we should not use extraordinary means of prolonging life or its semblance when, after careful consideration, consultation and the application of the most well conceived therapy it becomes apparent that there is no hope for the recovery of the patient....'

"Our decision in this case is consistent with the current medical ethos in this area.

"There is implicit recognition in the law of the Commonwealth, as elsewhere, that a person has a strong interest in being free from nonconsensual invasion of his bodily integrity....

"Of even broader import, but arising from the same regard for human dignity and self-determination, is the unwritten constitutional right of privacy found in penumbra of specific guaranties of the Bill of Rights.... As this constitutional guaranty reaches out to protect the freedom of a woman to terminate pregnancy under certain conditions...so it encompasses the right of a patient to preseve his or her right to privacy against unwanted infringements of bodily integrity in appropriate circumstances....

"The question when the circumstances are appropriate for the exercise of this privacy right depends on the proper identification of State interests. It is not surprising that courts have, in the course of investigating State interests in various medical contexts and under various formulations of the individual rights involved, reached differing views on the nature and the extent of State interests....

"As distilled from...cases, the State has claimed interest in: (1) the preservation of life; (2) the protection of the interests of innocent third parties; (3) the prevention of suicide; and (4) maintaining the ethical integrity of the medical profession.

"It is clear that the most significant of the asserted State interests is that of the preservation of human life. Recognition of such an interest, however, does not necessarily resolve the problem where the affliction or disease clearly indicates that life will soon, and inevitably, be extinguished. The interest of the State in prolonging a life must be reconciled with the interest of an individual to reject the traumatic cost of that prolongation. There is a substantial distinction in the State's insistence that human life be saved where the affliction is curable, as opposed to the State interest where, as here, the issue is not whether but when, for how long, and at what cost to the individual that life may be briefly extended. Even if we assume that the State has an additional interest in seeing to it that individual decisions on the prolongation of life do not in any way tend to 'cheapen' the value which is placed in the concept of living...we believe it is not inconsistent to recognize a right to decline medical treatment in a situation of incurable illness. The constitutional right to privacy, as we conceive it, is an expression of the sanctity of individual free life. The value of life as so perceived is lessened not by a decision to refuse treatment, but by the failure to allow a competent human being the right of choice.

"A second interest of considerable magnitude, which the State may have some interest in asserting, is that of protecting third parties, particularly minor children, from the emotional and financial damage which may occur as a result of the decision of a competent adult to refuse life-saving or life-prolonging treatment.... We need not reach this aspect of claimed State interest as it is not in issue on the facts of this case.

"The last State interest requiring discussion is that of the maintenance of the ethical integrity of the medical profession as well as allowing hospitals the full opportunity to care for people under their control....* Prevailing medical ethical practice does not, without ex-

---

*"The interest in protecting against suicide seems to require little if any discussion. In the case of the competent adult's refusing medical treatment such an act does not necessarily

→

ception, demand that all efforts toward life prolongation be made in all circumstances. Rather, as indicated in *Quinlan*, the prevailing ethical practice seems to be to recognize that the dying are more often in need of comfort than treatment. Recognition of the right to refuse necessary treatment in appropriate circumstances is consistent with existing medical mores; such a doctrine does not threaten either the integrity of the medical profession, the proper role of hospitals in caring for such patients or the State's interest in protecting the same....

"Applying the considerations discussed in this subsection to the decision made by the probate judge in the circumstances of the case before us, we are satisfied that his decision was consistent with a proper balancing of applicable State and individual interests....

***

"The best interests of an incompetent person are not necessarily served by imposing on such persons results not mandated as to competent persons similarly situated. It does not advance the interest of the State or the ward to treat the ward as a person of lesser status or dignity than others. To protect the incompetent person within its power, the State must recognize the dignity and worth of such a person and afford to that person the same panoply of rights and choices it recognizes in competent persons. If a competent person faced with death may choose to decline treatment which not only will not cure the person but which substantially may increase suffering in exchange for a possible yet brief prolongation of life, then it cannot be said that it is always in the 'best interests' of the ward to require submission to such treatment. Nor do statistical factors indicating that a majority of competent persons similarly situated choose treatment resolve the issue. The significant decisions of life are more complex than statistical determinations. Individual choice is determined not by the vote of the majority but by the complexities of the singular situation viewed from the unique perspective of the person called on to

---

constitute suicide since (1) in refusing treatment the patient may not have the specific intent to die, and (2) even if he did, to the extent that the cause of death was from natural causes the patient did not set the death producing agent in motion with the intent of causing his own death.... Furthermore, the underlying State interest in this area lies in the prevention of irrational self-destruction. What we consider here is a competent, rational decision to refuse treatment when death is inevitable and the treatment offers no hope of cure or preservation of life. There is no connection between the conduct here in issue and any State concern to prevent suicide...."

make the decision. To presume that the incompetent person must always be subjected to what many rational and intelligent persons may decline is to downgrade the status of the incompetent persons by placing a lesser value on his intrinsic human worth and vitality.

* * *

"...We believe that both the guardian *ad litem* in his recommendation and the judge in his decision should have attempted (as they did) to ascertain the incompetent person's actual interests and preferences. In short, the decision in cases such as this should be that which would be made by the incompetent person, if that person were competent, but taking into account the present and future incompetency of the individual as one of the factors which would necessarily enter into the decision–making process of the competent person. Having recognized the right of a competent person to make for himself the same decision as the court made in this case, the question is, do the facts on the record support the proposition that Saikewicz himself would have made the decision under the standard set forth? We believe they do.

"The two factors considered by the probate judge to weigh in favor of administering chemotherapy were: (1) the fact that most people elect chemotherapy and (2) the chance of a longer life. Both are appropriate indicators of what Saikewicz himself would have wanted, provided that due allowance is taken for this individual's present and future incompetency. We have already discussed the perspective this brings to the fact that most people choose to undergo chemotherapy. With regard to the second factor, the chance of a longer life carries the same weight for Saikewicz as for any other person, the value of life under the law having no relation to intelligence or social position. Intertwined with this consideration is the hope that a cure, temporary or permanent, will be discovered during the period of extra weeks or months potentially made available by chemotherapy. The guardian *ad litem* investigated this possibility and found no reason to hope for a dramatic breakthrough in the time frame relevant to the decision.

"The probate judge identified six factors weighing against administration of chemotherapy. Four of these — Saikewicz's age, and the probable side effects of treatment, the low chance of producing remission, and the certainty that treatment will cause immediate suffering—were clearly established by the medical testimony to be considerations that any individual would weigh carefully. A fifth factor—Saikewicz's inability to cooperate with the treatment—introduces those considerations that are unique to this individual and which therefore are essential to the proper exercise of substituted judgment. The judge heard testimony that Saikewicz would have no comprehension of the reasons for the severe disruption of his formerly secure and stable environment occasioned by the chemotherapy. He therefore would experience fear without the understanding from which other patients draw strength. The inability to anticipate and prepare for the severe side effects of the drugs leaves room only for confusion and disorientation. The possibility that such a naturally uncooperative patient would have to be physically restrained to allow the slow intravenous administration of drugs could only compound his pain and fear, as well as possibly jeopardize the ability of his body to withstand the toxic effects of the drugs.

"The sixth factor identified by the judge as weighing against chemotherapy was 'the quality of life possible for him even if the treatment does bring about remission.' To the extent that this formulation equates the value of life with any measure of the quality of life, we firmly reject it. A reading of the entire record clearly reveals, however, the judge's concern that special care be taken to respect the dignity and worth of Saikewicz's life precisely because of his vulnerable position. The judge, as well as all the parties, were keenly aware that the supposed ability of Saikewicz, by virtue of his mental retardation, to appreciate or experience life had no place in the decision before them. Rather than reading the judge's formulation in a manner that demeans the value of the life of one who is mentally retarded, the vague, and perhaps ill-chosen, term 'quality of life' should be understood as a reference to the continuing state of pain and disorientation precipitated by the chemotherapy treatment. Viewing the term in this manner, we are satisfied that the decision to withhold treatment from Saikewicz was based on a regard for his actual interests and preferences and that the facts supported this decision."

* * *

SATZ V. PERLMUTTER

(District Court of Appeal of Florida, 1978)
362 S. 2d 160

May a competent adult who suffers from a terminal disease exercise his right to die?

JUDGE LETTS:

* * *

"Seventy-three-year-old Abe Perlmutter lies mortally sick in a hospital, suffering from amyotrophic lateral sclerosis (Lou Gehrig's disease) diagnosed in January, 1977. There is no cure and normal life expectancy, from time of diagnosis, is but two years. In Mr. Perlmutter, the affliction has progressed to the point of virtual incapability of movement, inability to breathe without a mechanical respirator and his very speech is an extreme effort. Even with the respirator, the prognosis is death within a short time. Notwithstanding, he remains in command of his mental faculties and legally competent. He seeks, with full approval of his adult family, to have the respirator removed from his trachea, which act, according to his physician, based upon medical probability, would result in 'a reasonable life expectancy of less than one hour.' Mr. Perlmutter is fully aware of the inevitable result of such removal, yet has attempted to remove it himself (hospital personnel, activated by an alarm, reconnected it). He has repeatedly stated to his family, 'I'm miserable, take it out' and, at a bedside hearing, told the obviously concerned trial judge that whatever would be in store for him if the respirator were removed, 'It can't be worse than what I'm going through now.'

"Pursuant to all of the foregoing, and upon the petition of Mr. Perlmutter himself, the trial judge entered a detailed and thoughtful final judgment which included the following language:

'ORDERED AND ADJUDGED that Abe Perlmutter, in the exercise of his right of privacy, may remain in defendant hospital or leave said hospital, free of the mechanical respirator now attached to his body and all defendants and their staffs are restrained from interfering with Plaintiff's decision.'

"We agree with the trial judge.

"The State's position is that it (1) has an overriding duty to preserve life, and (2) that termination of supportive care, whether it be by the patient, his family or medical personnel, is an unlawful killing of a human being.... The hospital, and its doctors, while not insensitive to this tragedy, fear not only criminal prosecution if they aid in removal of the mechanical device, but also civil liability. In the absence of prior Florida law on the subject, their fears cannot be discounted.

"The pros and cons involved in such tragedies which bedevil contemporary society, mainly because of incredible advancement in scientific medicine, are all exhaustively discussed in *Superintendent of Belchertown v. Saikewicz*. As *Saikewicz* points out, the right of an individual to refuse medical treatment is tempered by the State's:

1. Interest in the preservation of life.
2. Need to protect innocent third parties.
3. Duty to prevent suicide.
4. Requirement that it help maintain the ethical integrity of medical practice.

"In the case at bar, none of these four considerations surmount the individual wishes of Abe Perlmutter. Thus we adopt the view of the line of cases discussed in *Saikewicz* which would allow Abe Perlmutter the right to refuse or discontinue treatment based upon 'the constitutional right to privacy...an expression of the sanctity of individual free choice and self-determination....' We would stress that this adoption is limited to the specific facts now before us, involving a competent adult patient....

* * *

"Moreover we find no requirement in the law that a competent, but otherwise mortally sick, patient undergo the surgery or treatment which constitutes the only hope for temporary prolongation of his life. This being so, we see little difference between a cancer-ridden patient who declines surgery, or chemotherapy, necessary for this temporary survival and the hopeless predicament which tragically afflicts Abe Perlmutter. It is true that the latter appears more drastic because, affirmatively, a mechanical device must be disconnected, as distinct from mere inaction. Notwithstanding, the principle is the same, for in both instances the hapless, but mentally competent, victim is choosing not to avail himself of one of the expensive marvels of modern medical science.

* * *

"There can be no doubt that the State does have an interest in preserving life, but...'there is a substantial distinction in the State's insistence that human life be saved where the affliction is curable, as opposed to the State interest where, as here, the issue is not whether, but when, for how long and at what cost to the individual (his) life may be briefly extended....' In the case at bar the condition is terminal, the patient's situation wretched and the continuation of his life temporary and totally artificial.

"Accordingly, we see no compelling State interest to interfere with Mr. Perlmutter's expressed wishes.

"...We point out that Abe Perlmutter is 73, his family adult and all in agreement with his wishes....

"As to suicide, the facts here unarguably reveal that Mr. Perlmutter would die, but for the respirator. The disconnecting of it, far from causing his unnatural death by means of a 'death-producing agent,' in fact will merely result in his death, if at all, from natural causes.... The testimony of Mr. Perlmutter...is that he really wants to live, but to do so, God and Mother Nature willing, under his own power. The basic wish to live, plus the fact that he did not self-induce his horrible affliction, precludes his further refusal of treatment being classed as attempted suicide.

"...We reach our conclusion that, because Abe Perlmutter has a right to refuse treatment in the first instance, he has a concomitant right to discontinue it.

"Lastly, as to the ethical integrity of medical practice, we again adopt the language of *Saikewicz*:

'...Prevailing medical ethical practice does not, without exception, demand that all efforts toward life prolongation be made in all circumstances. Rather,...the prevailing ethical practice seems to be to recognize that the dying are more often in need of comfort than treatment....'

"It is our conclusion, therefore, under the facts before us, that when these several public policy interests are weighted against the rights of Mr. Perlmutter, the latter must and should prevail. Abe Perlmutter should be allowed to make his choice to die with dignity, notwithstanding over a dozen legislative failures in this state to adopt suitable legislation in this field. It is all very convenient to insist on continuing Mr. Perlmutter's life so that there can be no question of foul play, no resulting civil liability and no possible trespass of medical ethics. However, it is quite another matter to do so at the patient's sole expense and against his competent will, thus inflicting never-ending physical torture on his body until the inevitable, but artificially suspended, moment of death. Such a source of conduct invades the patient's constitutional right of privacy, removes his freedom of choice and invades his right to self-determine."

***

(The separate concurring opinion of Judge Anstead is deleted.)

IN RE PHILLIP B.

(California Court of Appeal, 1979)
92 Cal. App. 3d 796

May a defective child be operated upon even if the parents refuse consent to the surgery?

CALDECOTT, PRESIDING JUSTICE:

***

"The petition requested that Phillip be declared a dependent child of the court for the special purpose of ensuring that he receive cardiac surgery for a congenital heart defect. Phillip's parents had refused to consent to the surgery. The juvenile court dismissed the petition. The appeal is from the order.

"Phillip is a 12-year-old boy suffering from Down's syndrome. At birth his parents decided he should live in a residential care facility. Phillip suffers from a congenital heart defect — a ventricular septal defect that results in elevated pulmonary blood pressure. Due to the defect, Phillip's heart must work three times harder than normal to supply blood to his body. When he over-exerts, unoxygenated blood travels the wrong way through the septal hole reaching his circulation, rather than the lungs.

"If the congenital heart defect is not corrected, damage to the lungs will increase to the point where his lungs will be unable to carry and oxygenate any blood. As a result, death follows. During the deterioration of the lungs, Phillip will suffer from a progressive loss of energy and vitality until he is forced to lead a bed-to-chair existence.

"Phillip's heart condition has been known since 1973. At that time Doctor Gathman, a pediatric cardiologist, examined Phillip and recommended cardiac catheterization to further define the anatomy and dynamics of Phillip's condition. Phillip's parents refused.

"In 1977, Doctor Gathman again recommended catheterization and this time Phillip's parents consented. The catheterization revealed the extensive nature of Phillip's septal defect, thus it was Doctor Gathman's recommendation that surgery be performed.

"Doctor Gathman referred Phillip to a second pediatric cardiologist, Doctor William French of Stanford Medical Center. Doctor French estimates the surgical mortality rate to be 5 to 10 percent, and notes that Down's syndrome children face a higher than average risk of postoperative complications. Doctor French found that Phillip's pulmonary vessels have already undergone some change from high pulmonary artery pressure. Without the operation, Phillip will begin to function less physically until he will be severely incapacitated. Doctor French agrees with Doctor Gathman that Phillip will enjoy a significant expansion of his life span if his defect is surgically corrected. Without surgery, Phillip may live at the outset 20 more years. Doctor French's opinion on the advisability of surgery was not asked.

"It is fundamental that parental autonomy is constitutionally protected. The United States Supreme Court has articulated the concept of personal liberty found in the Fourteenth Amendment as a right of privacy which extends to certain aspects of a family relationship....

"Inherent in the preference for parental autonomy is a commitment to diverse life-styles, including the right of parents to raise their children as they think best. Legal judgments regarding the value of childrearing patterns should be kept to a minimum so long as the child is afforded the best available opportunity to fulfill his potential in society.

"Parental autonomy, however, is not absolute. The state is the guardian of society's basic values. Under the doctrine of *parens patriae*, the state has a right, indeed, a duty, to protect children.... State officials may interfere in family matters to safeguard the child's health, educational development and emotional well-being.

"One of the most basic values protected by the state is the sanctity of human life.... Where parents fail to provide their children with adequate medical care, the state is justified to intervene. However, since the state should usually defer to the wishes of the parents, it has a serious burden of justification before abridging parental autonomy by substituting its judgment for that of the parents.

"Several relevant factors must be taken into consideration before a state insists upon medical treatment rejected by the parents. The state should examine the seriousness of the harm the child is suffering or the substantial likelihood that he will suffer harm; the evaluation for the treatment by the medical profession; the risks involved in medically treating the child; and the expressed preferences of the child. Of course, the underlying consideration is the child's welfare and whether his best interests will be served by the medical treatment.

***

"Turning to the facts of this case, one expert witness testified that Phillip's case was more risky than the average for two reasons. One, he has pulmonary vascular changes and statistically this would make the operation more risky in that he would be subject to more complications than if he did not have these changes. Two, children with Down's syndrome have more problems in the postoperative period. This witness put the mortality rate at 5 to 10 percent, and the morbidity would be somewhat higher. When asked if he knew of a case in which this type of operation had been performed on a Down's syndrome child, the witness replied that he did, but could not remember a case involving a child who had the degree of pulmonary vascular change that Phillip had. Another expert witness testified that one of the risks of surgery to correct a ventricular septal defect was damage to the nerve that controls the heartbeat as the nerve is in the same area as the defect. When this occurs a pacemaker would be required.

***

"On reading the record we can see the trial court's attempt to balance the possible benefits to be gained from the operation against the risks involved. The court had before it a child suffering not only from a ventricular septal defect but also from Down's syndrome, with its higher than average morbidity, and the presence of pulmonary vascular changes. In light of these facts, we cannot say as a matter of law that there was no substantial evidence to support the decision of the trial court.

***

"The order dismissing the petition is affirmed."

(Rattiger and Christian, J.J. concur. Mosk, J. dissented.)

APPLICATION OF CICERO

(Supreme Court, State of New York, 1979)
421 N.Y.S. 2d 965

In the absence of parental consent, can a court order surgery for a spina bifida baby?

MARTIN B. STECHER, JUSTICE:

***

" '...[Spina bifida with meningomyelocele] is evident at birth as a skin defect over the back, bordered laterally by bony prominences of the unfused neural arches of the vertebrae. The defect is usually covered by a transparent membrane which may have neural tissue attached to its inner surface.' Cerebrospinal fluid may accumulate under the membrane causing it to bulge. This is the condition with which the Vataj infant was born.

"Failure to repair the opening presents a danger of perforation, highly probable infection, such as spinal meningitis, and death. The likelihood of survival beyond the age of six months is poor, absent treatment. Treatment is recommended within forty-eight hours of birth. The membrane covering this child's lesion shows signs of progressive erosion making immediate surgery necessary.

"The parents have refused treatment and insist on taking the child home. Their attitude, as expressed by the child's father, is 'let God decide' if the child is to live or die. Their rejection of treatment does not appear to stem from the kind of religious conviction with which judges are often faced....

"Initially, the father consented to surgery but appears to have withdrawn that consent only when the potential enormity of this disorder was fully explained to him by the physicians.

* * *

"This is not a case where the court is asked to preserve an existence which cannot be a life. What is asked is that a child born with handicaps be given a reasonable opportunity to live, to grow and hopefully to surmount those handicaps. If the power to make that choice is vested in the court, there can be no doubt as to what the choice must be.

* * *

"The argument is made that by granting the petition the parental right to choose [sic] the treatment, upbringing and welfare of the child is infringed upon by the court....

"Parental rights, however, are not absolute. Children are not property whose disposition is left to parental discretion without hindrance.... Where the child's welfare demands judicial intervention, this court is empowered to intervene.... Certainly, every physician who prefers a course of treatment rejected by a parent is not privileged to have the court decide upon the treatment under its *parens patriae* powers....

"But where, as here, a child has a reasonable chance to live a useful, fulfilled life, the court will not permit parental inaction to deny that chance.

"There is a hint in this proceeding of a philosophy that newborn, 'hopeless' lives should be permitted to expire without an effort to save those lives. Fortunately, the medical evidence here is such that we do not confront a 'hopeless' life. As Justice Asch has pointed out, ...'(t)here is a strident cry in America to terminate the lives of *other* people — deemed physically or mentally defective....' This court was not constituted to heed that cry...."

* * *

MATTER OF STORAR
AND
MATTER OF EICHNER

(Court of Appeals, New York, 1981)
52 N.Y.S. 2d 266

In the Eichner case, Brother Fox was eighty-three years old and terminally ill. On numerous occasions he had expressed the view that he did not wish extreme measures to be taken to prolong his life. When he became comatose, his guardian sought to have life-sustaining medical treatment discontinued.

In Storar, a fifty-two-year-old profoundly retarded man developed terminal cancer. John Storar had a mental age of eighteen months and had been in a state institution since the age of five. His seventy-seven-year-old mother, however, remained close to her child and visited him almost daily. After a time, the mother refused to approve blood transfusions for her child. John Storar plainly disliked the transfusions, but after treatment he did show greater energy. The state sought permission to continue John Storar's blood transfusions.

JUDGE WACHTELER:

* * *

"...At common law, every person 'of adult years and sound mind has a right to determine what should be done with his own body; and a surgeon who performs an operation without his patient's consent commits an assault, for which he is liable in damages.... This is true except in cases of emergency where the patient is unconscious and where it is necessary to operate before consent can be obtained...' The basic right of a patient to control the course of his medical treatment has been recognized by the Legislature (see Public Health Law §2504, 2805-d; CPLR 4401-a).

"Father Eichner urges that this right is also guaranteed by the Constitution, as an aspect of the right to privacy.... The current law identifies the patient's right to determine the course of his own medical treatment as paramount to what might otherwise be the doctor's obligation to provide needed medical care. A State which imposes the civil liability on a doctor if he violates the patient's right cannot be held to have violated his legal or professional responsibilities when he honors the right of a competent adult patient to decline medical treatment.

"The District Attorney also urges that whatever right the patient may have is entirely personal and may not be exercised by a third party once the patient becomes incompetent. He notes that although a court may appoint a guardian to manage an incompetent's financial affairs and to supervise his person, some rights have been held to be too personal to be exercised by an incompetent's representative.

"...He argues that a right to decline lifesaving treatment conflicts with the patient's fundamental and constitutionally guaranteed right to life (U.S. Constitution, Fourteenth Amendment) and to permit a third party to choose between the two means, in effect, that the right to life is lost once the patient becomes incompetent. Finally he urges that if a patient's right to decline medical treatment survives his incompetency, it must yield to the State's overriding interest in prohibiting one person from causing the death of another, as is evidenced by the homicide laws.

* * *

"...Clear and convincing proof should also be required in cases where it is claimed that a person, now incompetent, left instructions to terminate life-sustaining procedures when there is no hope of recovery....

"In this case the proof was compelling. There was no suggestion that the witnesses who testified for the petitioner had any motive other than to see that Brother Fox' [sic] stated wishes were respected. The finding that he carefully reflected on the subject, expressed his views and concluded not to have his life prolonged by medical means if there were no hope of recovery is supported by his religious beliefs and is not inconsistent with his life of unselfish religious devotion. These were obviously solemn pronouncements and not casual remarks made at some social gathering, nor can it be said that he was too young to realize or feel the consequences of his statements.... That this was a persistent commitment is evidenced by the fact that he reiterated the decision but two months before his final hospitalization.... In sum, the evidence clearly and convincingly shows that Brother Fox did not want to be maintained in a vegetative coma by use of a respirator.

"...John Storar was never competent at any time in his life. He was always totally incapable of understanding or making reasoned decision about medical treatment. Thus it is unrealistic to attempt to determine whether he would want to continue potentially life-prolonging treatment if he were competent. As one of the experts testified at the hearing, that would be similar to asking whether 'if it snowed all summer would it then be winter?' Mentally John Storar was an infant and that is the only realistic way to assess his rights in this litigation....

"A parent or guardian has a right to consent to medical treatment on behalf of an infant.... The parent, however, may not deprive a child of life-saving treatment, however well intentioned.... Even when the parents' decision to decline necessary treatment is based on constitutional grounds, such as religious beliefs, it must yield to the State's interests, as *parens patriae*, in protecting the health and welfare of the child.... Of course it is not for the courts to determine the most 'effective' treatment when the parents have chosen among reasonable alternatives.... But the courts may not permit a parent to deny a child all treatment for a condition which threatens his life....

"In the Storar case there is the additional complication of two threats to his life. There was cancer of the bladder which was incurable and would in all probability claim his life. There was also the related loss of blood which posed the risk of an earlier death, but which, at least at the time of the hearing, could be replaced by transfusions. Thus, as one of the experts noted, the transfusions were analogous to food — they would not cure the cancer, but they could eliminate the risk of death from another treatable cause. Of course, John Storar did not like them, as might be expected of one with an infant's mentality. But the evidence convincingly shows that the transfusions did not involve excessive pain and that without them his mental and physical abilities would not be maintained at the usual level. With the transfusions on the other hand, he was essentially the same as he was before except of course he had a fatal illness which would ultimately claim his life. Thus, on the record, we have concluded that the application for permission to continue the transfusions should have been granted. Although we understand and respect his mother's despair, as we respect the beliefs of those who oppose transfusions on religious grounds, a court should not in the circumstances of this case allow an incompetent patient to bleed to death because someone, even someone as close as a parent or sibling, feels that this is best for one with an incurable disease."

***

JUDGE JONES DISSENTING IN PART:

***

"...We all recognize the right of a competent adult to make decisions with respect to his own medical or surgical care even if the consequence of the particular decision be to hasten death. The question before us is whether, and under what circumstances, a surrogate de-

cision can be made on behalf of the patient when he is incompetent
to make it himself, where he has been diagnosed as incurably ill, and
where the decision relates to the withholding or withdrawal of extraordinary life support medical procedures. The question poses the
problem of judicial involvement in passive euthanasia...the deliberate withholding or withdrawal of available clinical means for the
prolongation of the life of a patient for whom there is little or no
hope of recovery or survival. Treating as the subject does with irreversible decisions affecting life and death, we approach, and even
may be thought by some to trespass on, the domain of Providence.
Few areas of judicial activity present such awesome questions or demand greater judicial wisdom and restraint.

"I identify two aspects of the problem so fundamental as to call
for exposition by this court, neither of which receives express attention in the writing of the majority. The first is explicit acknowledgment that the problem is one which the judicial system is unsuited
and ill-equipped to solve and which should not usually be made the
subject of judicial attention. The lapse of time necessarily consumed
in appellate review before there can be a final judicial determination
will almost always be unacceptable and makes recourse to judicial
proceedings impractical. The methodology and the techniques for
our classic adversary system are not best suited to the resolution of
the issues presented. The courts can claim no particular competence
to reach the difficult ultimate decision, depending as it necessarily
must not only on medical data, but on theological tenets and perceptions of human values which defy classification and calibration.

"There is reliable information that for many years physicians and
members of patient's families, often in consultation with religious
counselors, have in actuality been making decisions to withhold or to
withdraw life-support procedures from incurably ill patients incapable of making the critical decisions for themselves. While, of course,
there can be no categorical assurance that there have been no erro-
neous decisions thus reached, or even that in isolated instances death
has not been unjustifiably hastened for unacceptable motives, at the
same time there is no empirical evidence that either society or its individual members have suffered significantly in consequence of the
absence of active judicial oversight. There is no indication that the
medical profession whose members are most closely aware of current
practices senses the need for or desires intervention.

"For all the foregoing reasons I would explicity affirm the proposition that judicial approval is not required for discontinuance of life-support procedures in situations such as those now before us and that neither civil nor criminal liability attaches simply by reason of the absence of a court order of authorization.

"As to the second aspect, I nevertheless recognize that there will be occasions in which the courts will have thrust on them cases such as the two now before us. It is not difficult to anticipate instances in which for one or more of a variety of reasons a member of the patient's family or a close friend might desire to seek formal judicial approval of a proposal to withhold or to withdraw a particular extraordinary life-support procedure. I would therefore explicitly affirm the authority of our courts, in proper cases and in proceedings appropriately instituted, to grant authorization for withholding or withdrawal of extraordinary life-support medical procedures, notwithstanding the absence of evidence of an anticipatory expression of the attitude or wishes of the particular patient....

"Thus, I would have hoped that our court in the appeals now before us, would expressly have recognized the availability of, but not the necessity for, judicial approval of surrogate decisions in cases such as these. The fact that there is no such recognition serves to underscore the high desirability, there and elsewhere expressed, of legislative attention and action.

* * *

"With respect to the disposition of the appeals in these two cases: as stated, I would concur in result in *Matter of Eichner*; in *Storar* I would modify the order of the Appellate Division to the extent of dismissing the petition of Charles S. Soper as Acting Director of the Newark Developmental Center, and, as so modified, affirm. The dismissal would be premised on lack of standing of the hospital (or its director on behalf of the hospital) as a medical care provider to have instituted the proceeding seeking judicial authorization to continue blood transfusions against the wishes of Dorothy Storar, the patient's mother, guardian and committee. Medical care providers have at best only a tangential interest in the outcome of the litigation and can have no legitimate individual stake in the institution (or continuation) or the discontinuance of the medical procedure.... Additionally I am apprehensive that to accord standing to medical care providers to seek authorization for continuation of extraordinary life-support procedures in cases such as this might foster a perception that obtaining judicial approval should be the normal expectation...and thus lead to an increase in the institution of such proceedings, in some instances as anticipatory defensive strategy with respect to possible future claims for malpractice. Nor would I know what significance, if any, to ascribe to the circumstances that extraordinary medical procedures in particular now often involve a very heavy economic cost which might at least, in some instances, have a bearing on the provider's incentive to institute or continue such care (as well, on the other side of the equation, as possibly to lead dependent family members to oppose expensive treatment). I would, however, recognize the standing of a member of the family such as John Storar's mother, or a close friend as in *Eichner*, to institute a judicial proceeding for authorization to withdraw life-support measures.

***

"While there was evidence to which the majority refers, that the discontinuation of blood transfusions would have 'eventually' led to John Storar's death (and inferentially perhaps before death would otherwise have been caused by his cancer of the bladder), no finding was made as to what extension of life would attend the continuation of transfusions. Supreme Court made the ambiguous finding, undisturbed by the Appellate Division, that 'Storar has a life expectancy of from two to six months regardless of whether the blood transfusions are continued or not.' Similarly, although evidence was introduced that following transfusions Storar had more energy and was able to resume most of his usual, limited activities, the courts below made no finding that continued transfusions would improve the quality of his life or, if so, in what respect or to what extent. In the absence of factual determinations with respect to these matters (and in my view the evidence in the record is not sufficient to justify this court's now supplying such findings as a matter of law), I cannot conclude as a matter of law that the courts below erred in authorizing discontinuance of the blood transfusions in light of the factual determinations which the courts did make, to wit:

That John had cancer of the bladder which was both inoperable and incurable, with a life expectancy of from two to six months; that one who has cancer of the bladder suffers severe pain and the need for medication increases as the cancer spreads; that John had been in frequent pain and as his pain had increased his need for medication had also increased;

That the blood transfusions were painful although not excessively so; that because of John's apprehension and manifest dislike of the procedure the nurse had been giving him a shot approximately one hour before the transfusion; that he submitted to the blood transfusions reluctantly and because of the force that compelled him to submit; that recently he had had to be physically restrained and to have his arm tied down to prevent him from pulling out the needle used for the transfusion; that in constrast to his behavior prior to the commencement of the transfusions, he thereafter ventured outside his room infrequently; that he had appeared to be progressively more uncomfortable during the procedures; that as a result of the transfusions there was frequent clotting in his urine which made urination more painful; that the blood contributed to increased levels of sensitivity to the pain he was experiencing and contributed to his discomfort;

That the transfusions did not serve to reduce John's pain or to make him more comfortable; that the blood forced on him did not serve a curative purpose or offer a reasonable hope of benefit;

That if the transfusions were stopped John would suffer no additional pain, his discomfort would not increase, and indeed cessation might serve to make him less aware of the physical sensations he was experiencing and even lead to a subsiding of the bleeding from his bladder lesions;

That in the circumstances the blood transfusions are extraordinary treatments;

That because of his lifelong profound mental retardation John was incompetent to refuse or consent to the continuation of the blood transfusions or to make a reasoned choice as to his own wishes or best interests;

That his mother over his lifetime had come to know and sense his wants and needs and was acutely sensitive to his best interests; that she had provided more love, personal care, and affection for John than any other person or institution, and was closer to feeling what John was feeling than anyone else; that his best interests were of crucial importance to her;

That in his mother's opinion it would have been in John's best interests to discontinue the transfusions, and she believed that he would wish to have them stopped.

"No one suggests that there is not sufficient evidence in this record to support each of these factual findings.

"I would hold that the courts below had power to authorize the withdrawal of extraordinary life-support measures and that, in the circumstances of this case, there was no error of law when the courts below exercised that power to grant Mrs. Storar's cross application to discontinue blood transfusions for her son, John."

***

(The dissenting opinion of Judge Fuchsberg is deleted.)

QUESTIONS

1. Is it easier for a court to recognize the right to die for an eighty-three-year-old man? Suppose Brother Fox was thirty years of age. Do you think his right to die would be so readily recognized?
2. How important are religious values in determining whether a right to die will be recognized? That is, suppose one's religion did not recognize such a right and when competent the patient had practiced that religion? Would it then be harder to recognize the right than in such cases as *Eichner* and *Quinlan* where there was not religious opposition to assertion of the right to die?
3. If a competent adult expresses a desire to exercise the right to die at a social gathering, should that be considered when that person is terminally ill and comatose? What would be the difference between that expression and one made by Brother Fox to his clerical colleagues? The difference between a statement at a social gathering and a signed "Living Will"?
4. Is the right to die a misnomer? Why not a right to live?

5. Should quality of life be considered in deciding whether or not the right to die should be exercised? If the patient is incompetent, should quality of life be considered in behalf of the patient? Would quality of life ever be good enough that an incompetent patient should not be allowed to die?

6. Who has the right to judge the quality of life? The State? Parents? Judges? Physicians? Competent patients? Incompetent patients?

7. Does the concept of right to die attack the view that all human life is sacred and should be preserved?

8. If a patient has no "Living Will" should it not be assumed that the patient wishes extreme measures to be taken to preserve life? After all, competent adults have the opportunity to make such a will. If they do not do so, are they not in effect saying that should they become incompetent and terminally ill they do not wish to exercise the right to die?

9. How is it possible under the concept of substituted judgment to determine the preferences of an incompetent patient, especially a patient who has always been incompetent?

CHAPTER 8

WRONGFUL LIFE

INTRODUCTION

THE essence of tort law is that persons may be sued and damages collected from them for harms done to others. The concept of wrongful life is an extension of the usual tort law concepts. If an infant is born with a serious defect, it can be argued that the parents are responsible for harming the infant. Had they undertaken reasonable measures, they would have been genetically screened, learned of the defective fetus, and aborted it. Instead, they brought a defective baby into the world. Given the severity of the defect, it would be argued in the infant's behalf that nonexistence was preferable to existence. If a court accepted this thesis, a child could collect damages from parents for the harm of being given life.

Steele states that courts have been very reluctant to recognize such claims. "However," he wrote, "disturbing signs among legal circles suggest that this judicial attitude may not always prevail."[1] Courts have been reluctant to recognize wrongful life claims for several reasons. The argument that one is done harm by being given life is a novel one, perhaps too much so for many judges. Additionally, courts have been unwilling to try to place a value on the damage of being born. How, for example, does one calculate the value of nonexistence and the costs of existence to arrive at an appropriate award? Courts are also reluctant to rule that human life can be so devoid of value that the meaninglessness of nonexistence is preferable. Since there is a fundamental right of reproductive privacy, it may also be that judges are unwilling to decide cases that could restrict that fundamental freedom.[2]

There has only been a slightly greater judicial willingness to award damages where wrongful-life suits are brought against per-

---

[1]Steele, Mark W.: Genetic screening and the public well being.In Hiller, Marc D. (Ed.):*Medical Ethics and the Law* (Cambridge, Mass., Ballinger Publishing Company, 1981, p. 858).
[2]Ibid., pp. 358-359.

sons other than parents of the defective child. Wrongful-life suits have, for example, been brought against physicians for failure to inform parents of the probability of giving birth to a defective child. If a woman has rubella early in pregnancy, her chances of giving birth to a defective child are about one in four. A wrongful-life case was brought against physicians for failure to warn the woman that rubella does pose such a danger.[3] Another example of wrongful-life suits against physicians involved Jewish parents who sued a physician on their child's behalf because the physician failed to test for Tay-Sachs disease. They argued that the probability was high enough that the physician should have attempted to determine if the fetus had Tay-Sachs disease. Had the physician so determined, the fetus would have been aborted.[4] Suits have also been brought against medical laboratories for erring in tests that would have warned parents that a fetus was defective and would have led them to seek an abortion.[5]

Wrongful-life suits against physicians or medical laboratories are often in conjunction with suits by parents for damages. While the infant sues for being born, the parents sue for the hardships and expense incurred by the birth of a defective child. The parents' argument is that they would not have suffered such hardship and expense if the physician or medical laboratory had not been negligent. Therefore, they are entitled to damages from the negligent party.

Wrongful-life suits are related to wrongful-birth suits, but they differ in that in a wrongful-birth suit it is not argued that nonexistence is preferable to existence. In wrongful-birth suits, such arguments are inappropriate because the baby is a healthy and normal child. A wrongful-birth suit might involve an unsuccessful sterilization where a husband was told that a vasectomy rendered him sterile. The birth of a healthy and normal child after an unexpected pregnancy can lead to a suit against the physician on grounds of misrepresentation, negligence, or breach of contract. In wrongful-birth cases, courts will often refuse to award damages on the grounds that no damages have been suffered, but that the unexpected child is a "blessing." Where damages are awarded, courts are reluctant

---

[3]*Gleitman v. Cosgrove*, 227 A. 2d 689 (1967).
[4]*Howard v. Lecher*, 297 N.Y.S. 2d 363 (1977).
[5]*Curlender v. Bio-Science Laboratories*, 165 Cal., Rptr. 477 (1980).

to make them for general damages caused by the birth of a child. Instead, damages will be for the financial impact of the child. Other courts have limited damages to costs of the failed sterilization procedure; costs of the pregnancy; pain and suffering associated with the pregnancy; and loss of consortium. Currently, wrongful-birth awards tend to be rather small and often do not include the expenses of raising the unexpected child.[6]

Wrongful-birth suits preceded wrongful-life suits and provided a useful foundation for them. Though wrongful-birth suits have been in the courts since 1934, it was not until 1963 that the courts dealt with the concept of wrongful life.[7] In that case, an illegitimate child sued his father for damages due to the stigma associated with illegitimacy.[8] The child's claim was that he should have never been born if birth would bring such stigma. The case, *Zepeda v. Zepeda,* did not result in an award of damages, primarily because the court feared an award would open the courts to massive numbers of suits. *Zepeda,* however, differed from later suits. In *Zepeda,* the child's life was less preferable than nonexistence because of the status of the child — its illegitimacy. In later cases, it was argued that a child's life was wrongful because of the child's incurable defects. In *Zepeda,* the father's marriage to the mother would have changed the status of the child and the quality of its life. Nothing, it was claimed in later cases, would make the child's life preferable to nonexistence.

---

[6]Greenfield, Vicki R.: Wrongful birth (*Journal of the American Medical Association, 248*:926-927, 1982); and Reilly, Philip R., and Milunsky, Aubrey: Medicolegal aspects of prenatal diagnosis. In Milunsky, Aubrey (Ed.):*Genetic Disorders and the Fetus* (New York, Plenum Press, 1979, pp. 611-619).
[7]Reilly and Milunsky, op cit., pp. 611-612.
[8]*Zepeda v. Zepeda,* 190 N.E. 2d 849 1963).

ZEPEDA V. ZEPEDA

(Appellate Court, State of Illinois, 1963)
190 N.E. 2d 849

May an illegitimate child sue his father for wrongful life?

JUDGE DIMPSEY:

* * *

"The plaintiff is the infant son of the defendant. He seeks damages from his father because he is an illegitimate child. He appeals from an order dismissing his suit and striking his complaint for its failure to state a cause of action.

* * *

"The factual averments of the complaint, which were admitted by the motion to strike, are: the defendant is the plaintiff's father; the defendant induced the plaintiff's mother to have sexual relations by promising to marry her; this promise was not kept and could not be kept because, unbeknown to the mother, the defendant was already married. The complaint charges that the promise was fraudulent, that the acts of the defendant were willful and that the defendant injured the plaintiff in his person, property and reputation by causing him to be born an adulterine bastard. The plaintiff seeks damages for the deprivation of this right to be a legitimate child, to have a normal home, to have a legal father, to inherit from his father, to inherit from his paternal ancestors and for being stigmatized as a bastard.

* * *

"We need not be concerned whether a tort was committed upon the mother by the defendant's false promise of marriage which induced her to have intercourse with him. Our problem is whether a tort was committed upon the child. Thus, the second question to confront us is, can a tort be inflicted upon a being simultaneously with its conception?

"The law of torts has been hesitant in recognizing what medical science has long known, that life begins at the moment of conception, and what theology has longer taught, that from the moment of conception every human being has the rights of a human person. Blackstone wrote that in the contemplation of the common law a child's life began when it 'is able to stir in the mother's womb....' Although other branches of the law, such as property and inheritance, recognized the legal existence of a child from conception, in tort a child was not a being separate from its mother until it was born. In the last few years a change has taken place in the law pertaining to prenatal physical injuries. From 1884 to 1946 it was universally held that under the common law there could be no recovery for such injuries.... There were occasional dissenting opinions; judges were troubled by the unfairness of holding that a child...was a human being from inheritance and property rights and not one if it suffered tortious physical injury. It was not until 1946 that a major breakthrough was made under the common law,...although one that received less attention had occurred in 1924.... Gradually thereafter various jurisdictions permitted actions from prenatal injuries if a child was viable at the time of injury and if it survived birth....

"The case at bar seems to be the natural result of the present course of the law permitting actions for physical injury ever closer to the moment of conception. In point of time it goes just a little further. The significance of this course to us is this: if recovery is to be permitted an infant injured one month after conception, why not if injured one week after, one minute after, or at the moment of conception? It is inevitable that the date will be further retrogressed. How can the law distinguish the day to day development of life? If there is human life, proved by subsequent birth, then that human life has the same rights at the time of conception as it has at any time thereafter. There cannot be absolutes in the minute to minute progress of life from sperm to ovum to cell, to embryo to fetus, to child.

"But what if the wrongful conduct takes place before conception? Can the defendant be held accountable if his act was completed before the plaintiff was conceived? Yes, for it is possible to incur, as Justice Holmes phrased it in the *Dietrich* case, 'a conditional prospective liability in tort to one not yet in being.' It makes no difference how much time elapses between a wrongful act and resulting injury if there is a causal relation between them....

"This brings us to the next question to be considered, the character of the plaintiff's injury. Injuries other than physical or to property are compensable in law.... The present complaint, however, does not charge mental distress....

"Likewise, the complaint does not state a cause of action for defamation....

"The plaintiff further complains of being deprived of the normal home that might have been his and of equality with the legitimate child he might have been. A legitimate child has the natural right to be wanted, loved and cared for. He also has an interest in preserving his family life and he may protect this interest against outside disturbance.... However, a legitimate child cannot maintain an action against his own parents for lack of affection, for failure to provide a pleasant home, for disrupting the family life or for being responsible for a divorce which has broken up the home. An illegitimate child cannot be given rights superior to those of a legitimate child, and the plaintiff has no cause of action on this account.

"But it would be pure fiction to say that the plaintiff suffers no injury. The lot of a child born out of wedlock, who is not adopted or legitimized, is a hard one....

* * *

"...Children born illegitimate have suffered an injury. If legitimation does not take place, the injury is continuous.If legitimation cannot take place, the injury is irreparable.

"The injury is not as tangible as a physical defect but it is as real. This is acknowledged by the State itself. The statutory provisions that a child's illegitimacy must be suppressed, in certain public records, is an admission of the hardship that can be caused by its disclosure. How often during his life does an illegitimate try to conceal his parentage and how often does he wince in shame when it is revealed? Public opinion may bring about more laws ameliorating further his legal status, but laws cannot temper the cruelty of those who hurl the epithet 'bastard' nor ease the bitterness in him who hears it, knowing it to be true. This, however, is but one phase, one manifestation of the basic injury, which is in being born and remaining an illegitimate. An illegitimate's very birth places him under a disability.

"It is of this that the plaintiff complains. His adulterine birth has placed him under a permanent disability. He protests not only the act which caused him to be born but birth itself. Love of life being

what it is, one may conjecture whether, if he were older, he would
feel the same way. As he grows from infancy to maturity the natural
instinct to preserve life may cause him to cherish his existence as
much as...he now deplores it. Be that as it may, the quintessence of
his complaint is that he was born and that he is....

***

"Recognition of the plaintiff's claim means creation of a new tort:
a cause of action for wrongful life. The legal implications of such a
tort are vast, the social impact could be staggering. If the new litigation were confined just to illegitimates it would be formidable. In
1968 there were 224,338 illegitimate births in the United States,
14,262 in Illinois and 10,182 in Chicago.... Not only are there more
such births year after year...but the ratio between illegitimate and legitimate births is increasing....

"That the doors of litigation would be opened wider might make
us proceed cautiously in approving a new action, but it would not
deter us. The plaintiff's claim cannot be rejected because there may
be others of equal merit. It is not the suits of illegitimates which give
us concern, great in numbers as these may be. What does disturb us
is the nature of the new action and the related suits which would be
encouraged. Encouragement would extend to all others born into
the world under conditions they might regard as adverse. One might
seek damages for being born of a certain color, another because of
race; one for being born with a hereditary disease, another for in-
heriting unfortunate family characteristics; one for being born into a
large and destitute family, another because a parent has an unsavory
reputation.

"The present case could be just a forerunner of those which may
confront the courts in the future. Without stimulating them, we may
have suits for wrongful life just as we now have for wrongful
death....

***

"If we are to have a legal action for such a radical concept as
wrongful life, it should come after thorough study of the consequences. This would be so even if the new action were to be restricted to illegitimates or even adulterine illegitimates. A study, of
the depth and scope warranted by the gravity of this action,

can best be made by the General Assembly which, as we have seen, has been steadily whittling away at the legal handicap shackling bastards and has given them rights almost equivalent to those born legitimate. Changing economic, social or political conditions, or scientific advancements, produce new problems which are constantly thrust upon the courts. These problems often require the remolding of the law, the extension of old remedies or the creation of new and instant remedies — but no recent development is presented by this case which demands an immediate remedy to keep abreast of progress. Although the legal questions unfolded are new, the problem is not; the social conditions producing the problem have existed since the advent of man.

"We have decided to affirm the dismissal of the complaint. We do this, despite our designation of the wrong committed herein as a tort, because of our belief that lawmaking, while inherent in the judicial process, should not be indulged in where the result could be as sweeping as here. The interest of society is so involved, the action needed to redress the tort could be so far-reaching, that the policy of the State should be declared by the representatives of the people.

"Affirmed."

GLEITMAN V. COSGROVE

(Supreme Court of New Jersey, 1967)

227 A. 2d 689

May a child collect damages from a doctor on the grounds that had the doctor informed its mother of the possible effects of German measles, it would have been aborted and therefore would not have suffered from severe birth defects? May the parents collect damages for the wrongful life of their child?

PROCTOR, J.:

* * *

"The first count of the complaint is on behalf of Jeffrey Gleitman, an infant, for his birth defects. The second count is by his mother, Sandra Gleitman, for the effects on her emotional state caused by her son's condition. And the third count is by his father, Irwin Gleitman, for the costs incurred in caring for Jeffrey. Defendants, Robert Cosgrove, Jr., and Jerome Dolan, are physicians specializing in obstetrics and gynecology engaged together in the practice of medicine in Jersey City.

"Sandra Gleitman consulted defendants on April 20, 1959. She was examined by Doctor Robert Cosgrove, Jr., and found by him to be two months pregnant. She informed him that on or about March 20, 1959 she had had an illness diagnosed as German measles. Mrs. Gleitman testified that Doctor Cosgrove, on receipt of this information and on inquiry by her, told her that the German measles would have no effect at all on her child.

"For the next three months Mrs. Gleitman received her prenatal medical care from the army doctors at Fort Gordon, Georgia where her husband was stationed. She informed the army doctors about the German measles she had had in her early pregnancy, and they instructed her to ask her regular physician about this when she returned home.

"She next consulted the defendants in July at which time she saw Doctor Dolan. Mrs. Gleitman testified that she repeated her inquiry about the effects of German measles and again received a reassuring answer. These inquiries and answers occurred on each of her subsequent visits.

"On November 25, 1959, Mrs. Gleitman was delivered of a boy, Jeffrey, at the Margaret Hague Maternity Hospital in Jersey City. Although at first the baby seemed normal, a few weeks later the substantial defects which Jeffrey has in sight, hearing, and speech began to become apparent. He has had several operations which have given him some visual capacity, and he attends a special correctional institute for blind and deaf children. His physical condition, which is seriously impaired, is not in dispute on this appeal.

"Plaintiffs' medical expert, Doctor Louis Fraulo, gave his opinion that Jeffrey's condition was causally related to the viral disease of German measles which Mrs. Gleitman had in March. Doctor Fraulo testified that women who have German measles in the first trimester of their pregnancy will produce infants with birth defects in 20 to 50 percent of the cases. Doctor Fraulo further stated that a physician who finds pregnancy and is given a history of German measles occurring during the term of pregnancy should inform his female patient of the likelihood of birth defects. In answer to a hypothetical question based on Mrs. Gleitman's testimony, Doctor Fraulo stated that defendants had deviated from generally accepted medical standards by not informing their pregnant patient of the likelihood of birth defects. A patient so informed, Doctor Fraulo testified, should then decide whether to bear the baby or have the pregnancy terminated by an abortion.

"Doctor Robert Cosgrove, Jr., agreed that Mrs. Gleitman had consulted him for her pregnancy on April 20, 1959 and had thereafter been the patient of Doctor Dolan and himself until November 25, 1959 when Jeffrey was born. He further agreed that the history given him had included the illness of German measles in March, and acknowledged that his duty as a physician required him to inform his patient of the possibility of birth defects. He testified, however, that in the presence of Doctor Samuel Cosgrove, since deceased, and a woman who appeared to be the mother of Mrs. Gleitman, he told his patient of a 20 percent chance her baby would have some defect. He also stated that he informed her that some doctors would recommend and perform an abortion for this reason, but that he did not think it proper to destroy four healthy babies because the fifth one would have some defect.

"Doctor Dolan testified that Mrs. Gleitman, whom he first saw in July when in any event it was too far along in the pregnancy for a medically safe abortion, had never asked him about the effects of German measles, and that he had never mentioned these effects to her. Doctor Dolan, as well as Doctor Edward C. Waters, who was called as an expert for the defendants, agreed that a physician had the duty of informing his patient as to the likelihood of birth defects which they both estimated would occur in some 20 to 25 percent of the cases where a female has German measles in the first trimester of her pregnancy.

"The theory of plaintiffs' suit is that defendants negligently failed to inform Mrs. Gleitman, their patient, of the effects which German measles might have upon the infant then in gestation. Had the mother been so informed, plaintiffs assert, she might have obtained other medical advice with a view to the obtaining of an abortion. Plaintiffs do not assert that Mrs. Gleitman's life or health was in jeopardy during the term of her pregnancy.

"As noted above the trial judge dismissed the three counts without submitting any of them to the jury. The claim of infant plaintiff was dismissed for failure to show that acts of the defendants were the proximate cause of Jeffrey's condition, and the claims by his mother and father were dismissed because the trial judge believed the suggested abortion would be criminal in New Jersey.

"Because the complaint was dismissed on motion for judgment by defendants, the testimony on behalf of plaintiffs together with all reasonable inferences therefrom will be assumed to be true. The motion for judgment of dismissal conceded for purposes of the motion the truth of plaintiffs' evidence.... Specifically, on this appeal we must take it to be the fact that Doctor Cosgrove, Jr., affirmatively misled Mrs.Gleitman on April 20, 1959 by telling her that the German measles she had in March would have no effect at all on her child then in gestation (despite the conflict in the evidence on this point).

"From our discussion of this case we will assume that somehow or somewhere Mrs. Gleitman could have obtained an abortion that would not have subjected participants to criminal sanctions, and that she did not do so because she relied on the incorrect advice of the defendant.

"At the outset it must be clearly understood that there is no suggestion by plaintiffs that defendants could have ordered any therapy—whether surgery, drugs or otherwise—which would have decreased the possibility that the infant then in gestation would be born with birth defects. The present case is sharply different from those cases where a deviation from standard medical practice affects the chances that an infant will be born with birth defects....

"The right of an infant to sue for prenatal torts was established in this state by *Smith v. Brennan*...where a child in gestation received injuries when his mother was in an automobile accident.... An essential part of the cause for action set forth in *Smith v. Brennan* is the 'disruption' or proximate cause of injury by act of commission or omission which results in impairment to what otherwise would be a normal healthy child. In the present case there is no contention that anything the defendants could have done would have decreased the likelihood that the infant would be born with defects. The condition of defendants was not the cause of infant plaintiff's condition.

"The infant plaintiff is therefore required to say not that he should have been born without defects but that he should not have been born at all. In the language of tort law he says: but for the negligence of defendants, he would not have been born to suffer with an impaired body. In other words, he claims that the conduct of defendants prevented his mother from obtaining an abortion which could have terminated his existence, and that his very life is 'wrongful.'

"The normal measure of damages in tort actions is compensatory. Damages are measured by comparing the condition plaintiff would have been in, had the defendants not been negligent, with plaintiff's impaired condition as a result of the negligence. The infant plaintiff would have us measure the difference between his life with defects against the utter void of nonexistence, but it is impossible to make such a determination. This Court cannot weight the value of life with impairments against the nonexistence of life itself. By asserting that he should not have been born, the infant plaintiff makes it logically impossible for a court to measure his alleged damages because of the impossibility of making the comparison required by compensatory remedies....

"We hold that the first count of the complaint on behalf of Jeffrey Gleitman is not actionable because the conduct complained of, even if true, does not give rise to damages cognizable at law.

"The mother and father stand in a somewhat different position from the infant. They are equally subject to the factual circumstances that no act by the defendants could have decreased the likelihood that the infant would be defective. However, Mrs. Gleitman can say that an abortion would have freed her of the emotional problems caused by the raising of a child with birth defects; and Mr. Gleitman can assert that it would have been less expensive for him to abort rather than raise the child. A considerable problem is raised by the claim of injury to the parents. In order to determine their compensatory damages a court would have to evaluate the denial to them of the intangible, unmeasurable, and complex human benefits of motherhood and fatherhood and weigh these against the alleged emotion and money injuries. Such a proposed weighing is similar to that which we have found impossible to perform for the infant plaintiff. When the parents say their child should not have been born, they make it impossible for a court to measure their damages in being the mother and father of a defective child.

"Denial of the claim for damages by adult plaintiffs is also required by a close look at exactly what it is they are here seeking. The thrust of their complaint is that they were denied the opportunity to terminate the life of their child while he was an embryo. Even under our assumption that an abortion could have been obtained without making its participants liable to criminal sanctions, substantial policy reasons prevent this Court from allowing tort damages for the denial of the opportunity to take an embryonic life.

"It is basic to the human condition to seek life and hold on to it however heavily burdened. If Jeffrey could have been asked as to whether his life should be snuffed out before his full term of gestation could run its course, our felt intuition of human nature tells us that he would almost surely choose life with defects as against no life at all....

"The right to life is inalienable in our society. A court cannot say what defects should prevent an embryo from being allowed life such that denial of the opportunity to terminate the existence of a defective child in embryo can support a cause for action. Examples of famous persons who have had great achievement despite physical defects come readily to mind, and many of us can think of examples close to home. A child need not be perfect to have a worthwhile life.

"We are not faced with the necessity of balancing the mother's life against that of her child. The sanctity of the single human life is the decisive factor in this suit in tort. Eugenic considerations are not controlling. We are not talking here about the breeding of prize cattle. It may have been easier for the mother and less expensive for the father to have terminated the life of their child while he was an embryo, but these alleged detriments cannot stand against the preciousness of the single human life to support a remedy in tort....

"Though we sympathize with the unfortunate situation in which these parents find themselves, we firmly believe the right of their child to live is greater than and precludes their right not to endure emotional and financial injury. We hold therefore that the second and third counts of the complaint are not actionable because the conduct complained of, even if true, does not give rise to damages cognizable at law; and even if such alleged damages were cognizable, a claim for them would be precluded by the countervailing public policy supporting the preciousness of human life.

* * *

"For the foregoing reasons the judgment of the trial court dismissing the three counts of the complaint is affirmed."

***

JUSTICE JACOBS, JOINED BY JUSTICE SCHETTING, DISSENTING:

"When Mrs. Gleitman told her obstetricians that she had German measles (rubella), they were placed under a clear duty to tell her of its high incidence of abnormal birth. That duty was not only a moral one but a legal one as well.... If the duty had been discharged, Mrs. Gleitman could have been safely and lawfully aborted and have been free to conceive again and give birth to a normal child. Instead she was told, according to her testimony which the majority assumes for the present purposes to be true, that her child would not be at all affected. In reliance on that she permitted the pregnancy to proceed and gave birth to a child who is almost blind, is deaf and mute and is probably mentally retarded. While the law cannot remove the heartache or undo the harm, it can afford some reasonable measure of compensation towards alleviating the financial burdens. In declining to do so, it permits a wrong with serious consequential injury to go wholly unredressed. That provides no deterrent to professional irresponsibility and is neither just nor compatible with expanding principles of liability in the field of torts.

"While the wrong was done directly to Mrs. Gleitman, in truth and reality it vitally affected her entire immediate family. Her husband's standing and injury alongside her should be self-evident since he was intimately concerned with the pregnancy and its consequences as was his wife.... And while logical objection may be advanced to the child's standing and injury, logic is not the determinative factor and should not be permitted to obscure that he has to bear the frightful weight of his abnormality throughout life, and that such compensation as is received from the defendants or either of them should be dedicated primarily to his care and the lessening of his difficulties. Indeed, if this were suitably provided for in the ultimate judgment, the technical presence or absence of the child as an additional party plaintiff would have little significance.

"I find no substantial basis for the majority's notion that it would be 'impossible' for the court or jury to deal properly with the matter of compensatory damages. The plaintiffs' thesis, which a jury could reasonably accept, is that, were it not for the breach of duty, the pregnancy would have been lawfully terminated and the plaintiffs would have been spared not only the incalculable emotional distress but also the readily measurable medical and maintenance expenses causally related to the abnormality. Surely a judicial system engaged daily in evaluating such matters as pain and suffering, which admittedly have 'no known dimensions, mathematical or financial' ...should be able to evaluate the harm which proximately resulted from the breach of duty. Indeed, even if there were more evaluation complexities than are truly present here, they would not furnish any sound basis for the total denial of recovery.

"The majority rests its rejection of the plaintiffs' action not only on its expressed difficulties with damages but also on its views as to the State's 'public policy.' But there is no policy favoring the breach of duty here or its immunization. Nor is there any dispute that the Gleitmans could have terminated the pregnancy lawfully outside New Jersey, at least in some foreign country. While the majority does not pass on the issue, I believe that the pregnancy could also have been terminated lawfully within New Jersey...."

***

(The concurring opinion by Justice Francis is deleted as is the partial dissent by Chief Justice Weintraub.)

BECKER V. SCHWARTZ

(Court of Appeals of New York, 1978)
386 N.E. 2d 887

Is a wrongful life claim justiciable?

JASON, JUDGE:

***

"...Delores Becker, then thirty-seven years of age, conceived a child in September, 1974. After Delores and her husband, Arnold Becker, learned of the pregnancy in October, they engaged the services of defendants, specialists in the field of obstetrics and gynecology. Thereafter, from approximately the tenth week of pregnancy until the birth of their child, Dolores Becker remained under defendant's exclusive care. Tragically, on May 10, 1975, Dolores Becker gave birth to a retarded and brain-damaged infant who suffers, and will continue to suffer for the remainder of her life, from Down's syndrome, commonly known as mongolism.

"It is the plaintiff's contention that throughout the period during which Dolores Becker was under the care of defendants, plaintiffs were never advised by defendants of the increased risk of Down's syndrome in children born to women over thirty-five years of age. Nor were they advised, allege plaintiffs, of the availability of an amniocentesis test to determine whether the fetus carried by Dolores Becker would be born with Down's syndrome.

"Plaintiffs commenced this action seeking damages on behalf of the infant for 'wrongful life,' and, in their own right, for the various sums of money they will be forced to expend for the long-term institutional care of their retarded child. Plaintiffs' complaint also seeks damages for the emotional and physical injury suffered by Dolores Becker as a result of the birth of her child, as well as damages for the injury suffered by Arnold Becker occasioned by the loss of his wife's services and the medical expenses stemming from her treatment.

***

"In the companion case, *Park v. Chessin*, Hetty Park gave birth in June, 1969 to a baby who, afflicted with polycystic kidney disease, died only five hours after birth. Concerned with a possible reoccurrence of this disease in a child conceived in the future, Hetty Park and her husband, Steven Park, consulted defendants, the obstetricians who treated Hetty Park during her first pregnancy, to determine the likelihood of this contingency. In response to plaintiffs' inquiry defendants are alleged to have informed plaintiffs that inasmuch as polycystic kidney disease was not hereditary, the chances of their conceiving a second child afflicted with this disease were 'practically nil.' Based upon this information, plaintiffs alleged that they exercised a conscious choice to seek conception of a second child. As a result, Hetty Park again became pregnant and gave birth in July, 1978 to a child who similarly suffered from polycystic kidney disease. Unlike their first child, however, plaintiffs' second child survived for two-and-one-half years before succumbing to this progressive disease.

"Alleging that contrary to defendants' advice polycystic kidney disease is in fact an inherited condition, and that had they been correctly informed of the true risk of reoccurrence of this disease in a second child, they would not have chosen to conceive, plaintiffs commenced this action seeking damages on behalf of the infant for 'wrongful life' and, in their own right, for the pecuniary expense they have borne for the care and treatment of their child until her death. Plaintiffs' complaint also seeks damages for the emotional and physical injuries suffered by Hetty Park as the result of the birth of her child; damages for emotional injuries and expenses suffered by Steven Park; damages for the injury suffered by Steven Park occasioned by the loss of his wife's services; and damages on behalf of plaintiffs, as administrators of their child's estate, for wrongful death.

* * *

"At the outset, emphasis must necessarily be placed upon the posture in which these cases are now before this court. The question presented for review is not whether plaintiffs should ultimately prevail in this litigation, but rather, more narrowly whether their complaints state cognizable causes of action. For the purposes of our review, limited as it is to an evaluation of the sufficiency of plaintiffs' complaints, their allegations must be assumed to be true.

* * *

"However, there are two flaws in plaintiffs' claims on behalf of their infants for wrongful life. The first, in a sense the more fundamental, is that is does not appear that the infants suffered any legally cognizable injury.... There is no precedent for recognition at the Appellate Division of 'the fundamental right of a child to be born as a whole, functional human being....' Whether it is better never to have been born at all than to have been born with even gross deficiencies is a mystery more properly to be left to the philosophers and the theologians.

"Surely the law can assert no competence to resolve the issue, particularly in view of the very nearly uniform high value which the law and mankind has placed on human life, rather than its absence. Not only is there to be found no predicate at common law or in statutory enactment for judicial recognition of the birth of a defective child as an injury to the child; the implications of any such proposition are staggering. Would claims be honored, assuming the breach of an identifiable duty, for less than a perfect birth? And by what standard or by whom would perfection be defined?

"There is also a second flaw. The remedy afforded an injured party in negligence is designed to place that party in the position he would have occupied but for the negligence of the defendant.... Thus, the damages recoverable on behalf of an infant for wrongful life are limited to that which is necessary to restore the infant to the position he or she would have occupied were it not for the failure of the defendant to render advice to the infant's parents in a nonnegligent manner. The theoretical hurdle to an assertion of damages on behalf of an infant accruing from a defendant's negligence in such a case becomes at once apparent. The very allegations of the complaint state that had the defendant not been negligent, the infant's parents would have chosen not to conceive, or, having conceived, to have terminated rather than to have carried the pregnancy to term, thereby depriving the infant plaintiff of his or her very existence. Simply put, a cause of action brought on behalf of an infant seeking recovery for wrongful life demands a calculation of damages dependent upon a comparison between the Hobson's choice of life in an impaired state and nonexistence. This comparison the law is not equipped to make.... Accordingly, plaintiffs' complaints insofar as they seek damages on behalf of their infants for wrongful life should be dismissed for failure to state a legally cognizable cause of action.

"There remains for consideration, however, the validity of plaintiffs' causes of action brought in their own right for damages accruing as a consequence of the birth of their infants. There can be no dispute at this stage of the pleadings that plaintiffs have alleged the existence of a duty flowing from defendants to themselves and that the breach of that duty was the proximate cause of the birth of their infants. That they have been damaged by the alleged negligence of defendants has also been pleaded. Unlike the causes of action brought on behalf of their infants for wrongful life, plaintiffs' causes of action also founded essentially upon a theory of negligence or medical malpractice, do allege ascertainable damages: the pecuniary expense which they have borne, and in *Becker* must continue to bear, for the care and treatment of their infants. Certainly, assuming the validity of plaintiffs' allegations, it can be said in traditional tort language that but for the defendants' breach of their duty to advise plaintiffs, the latter would not have been required to assume these obligations. Calculation of damages necessary to make plaintiffs whole in relation to these expenditures requires nothing extraordinary....

"Of course, this is not to say that plaintiffs may recover for psychic or emotional harm alleged to have occurred as a consequence of the birth of their infants in an impaired state....

* * *

"...[P]arents of a deformed infant will suffer the anguish that only parents can experience upon the birth of a child in an impaired state. However, notwithstanding the birth of a child afflicted with an abnormality, and certainly dependent upon the extent of the affliction, parents may yet experience a love that even an abnormality cannot fully dampen. To assess damage for emotional harm endured by the parents of such a child would, in all fairness, require consideration of this factor in mitigation of the parents' emotional injuries.... [U]nlike plaintiffs' causes of action for pecuniary loss in the instant cases, calculation of damages for plaintiffs' emotional injuries remains too speculative to permit recovery notwithstanding the breach of a duty flowing from the defendant to themselves. As in the case of plaintiffs' causes of action for damages on behalf of their infants for wrongful life, the cognizability of their actions for emotional harm is a question best left for legislative address."

* * *

FUCHSBERG, JUDGE (CONCURRING):

"...Who then can say, as it was essential to the parents' causes of action that they say for themselves, that, had it been possible to make the risk known to the children-to-be — in their cellular or fetal state, or let us say, in the mind's eye of their future parents — that the children too would have preferred that they not be born at all?

"To ordinary mortals, the answer to the question obviously is 'no one.' Certainly the answer does not lie in the exercise of the children, if their mental conditions permit, of subjective judgments long after their births. Therefore, whatever be the metaphysical or philosophical answer — speculative, perhaps debatable, but hardly resolvable —

and however desirable it may be for society to otherwise treat these problems with sensitivity, I am compelled to conclude that the matter is just not justiciable....'"

***

WACHTLER, JUDGE (DISSENTING IN PART):

"Insofar as this opinion relates to the case of *Becker v. Schwartz*, I agree with the majority that the suit for 'wrongful life' brought on behalf of the infant should be dismissed. I would, however, also dismiss the parents' collateral suit for the expense of rearing an unwanted child.

"A doctor who provides prenatal care to an expectant mother should not be held liable if the child is born with a genetic defect. Any attempt to find the physician responsible, even to a limited extent, for an injury which the child unquestionably inherited from his parents, requires a distortion or abandonment of fundamental legal principles and recognition, by the courts, of controversial rights and duties more appropriate for consideration and debate by a legislative body. These problems, which are always present when the child born with a genetic disorder seeks to hold the doctor responsible, are compounded when the parents seek compensation, on their own behalf, for collateral injuries occasioned by emotional distress or the increased cost of caring for a handicapped child.

"The heart of the problem in these cases is that the physician cannot be said to have caused the defect. The disorder is genetic and not the result of any injury negligently inflicted by the doctor. In addition, it is incurable and was incurable from the moment of conception. Thus, the doctor's alleged negligent failure to detect it during a prenatal examination cannot be considered a cause of the condition by analogy to those cases in which the doctor has failed to make a timely diagnosis of a curable disease. The child's handicap is an inexorable result of conception and birth.

"...Even if we assume, as we must on a motion to dismiss the complaint, that the parents would have made all the difficult decisions leading to an abortion — a conclusion which could be certain, if ever, only in retrospect — we must still go to great lengths to find that the doctors, failure to detect the defect was the cause, indeed the proximate cause, of the child's handicapped life. And the causal relationship is even more remote when the parents seek to recover for an injury they have suffered as a result of the alleged injury to the child.

"But the problems extend beyond causation. There is also the question as to what right the doctor violated and to whom the right belongs. The infant essentially claims that she had a right not to be born when birth would necessarily mean a life of hardship. The majority notes that the damages for violation of such a right would be impossible to assess. But on an even more fundamental level this cause of action must fail because the courts have long refused to recognize that such a right exists....

"...[T]here is no right not be born, even into a life of hardship, and thus no right cognizable at law which the defendant can be said to have violated.

"Since the infant's suit must be dismissed, the parents' cause of action for the costs of 'special treatment, teaching care, medical services, aid and assistance throughout the lifetime of the infant' should be dismissed as well. A parent's right to recover expenses occasioned by an injury to the child 'is based upon and arises out of the negligence which causes the injury to the child....' If the child cannot establish a good cause of action to recover for its injury, the parents' suit for collateral losses, flowing from the injury to the child, must also fail....

* * *

"In sum, by holding the doctor responsible for the birth of a genetically handicapped child, and thus obligated to pay most, if not all, of the costs of lifetime care and support, the court has created a kind of medical paternity suit. It is a tort without precedent, and at variance with existing precedents old and new. Indeed the members of the majority are divided among themselves as to what principle of law requires the doctor to pay damages in this cause. The limits of this new liability cannot be predicated. But if it is to be limited at all it would appear that it can only be confined by drawing arbitrary and artificial boundaries which a majority of the court consider popular or desirable. This alone should be sufficient to indicate that these cases pose a problem which can only be properly resolved by a legislative body, and not by courts of law."

* * *

(In reference to Becker v. Schwartz, Judge Gabrielli concurred in part and dissented in part for the reasons given by Judge Wachtler. Judge Cooke joined in Judge Fuchsberg's concurring opinion. In reference to Park v. Chessin, Judge Cooke joined in Judge Fuschberg's concurrence. Judge Wachteler took no part in the case. Judge Gabrielli concurred in part and dissented in part.)

TURPIN V. SORTINI

(Supreme Court of California, 1982)
643 P. 2d 954

To what extent may a child recover damages for wrongful life?

KAUS, JUSTICE:

* * *

"The allegations of the complaint disclose the following facts. On September 24, 1976, James and Donna Turpin, acting on the advice of their pediatrician, brought their first — and at that time their only — daughter, Hope, to the Leon S. Peters Rehabilitation Center at the Fresno Community Hospital for evaluation of a possible hearing defect. Hope was examined and tested by Adam J. Sortini, a licensed professional specializing in the diagnosis and treatment of speech and hearing defects.

"The complaint alleges that Sortini and other persons at the hospital negligently examined, tested and evaluated Hope and incorrectly advised her pediatrician that her hearing was within normal limits when, in reality, she was 'stone deaf' as a result of a hereditary ailment. Hope's parents did not learn of her condition until October 15, 1977 when it was diagnosed by other specialists. According to the complaint, the nature of the condition is such that there is a 'reasonable degree of medical probability' that the hearing defect would be inherited by any offspring of James and Donna.

"The complaint further alleges that in December, 1976, before learning of Hope's true condition and relying on defendants' diagnosis, James and Donna conceived a second child, Joy. The complaint avers that had the Turpins known of Hope's hereditary deafness they would not have conceived Joy. Joy was born August 23, 1977 and suffers from the same total deafness as Hope.

"...[T]he only cause before us on this appeal...was brought on behalf of Joy and seeks (1) general damages for being 'deprived of the fundamental right of a child to be born as a whole, functional human being without total deafness' and (2) special damages for the 'extraordinary expenses for specialized teaching, training and hearing equipment' which she will incur during her lifetime as a result of her hearing impairment....

* * *

"A plaintiff's remedy in tort is compensatory in nature and damages are generally intended not to punish a negligent defendant but to restore an injured person as nearly as possible to the position he or she would have been in had the wrong not been done. Because nothing defendants could have done would have given plaintiff an unimpaired life, it appears inconsistent with basic tort principles to view the injury for which defendants are legally responsible solely by reference to plaintiff's present condition without taking into consideration the fact that if defendants had not been negligent she would not have been born at all....

"If the relevant injury in this case is the change in the plaintiff's position attributable to the tortfeasor's actions, then the injury which plaintiff has suffered is that, as a result of defendants' negligence, she has been born with a hereditary ailment rather than not being born at all. Although plaintiff has not phrased her claim for general damages in these terms, most courts and commentators have recognized that the basic claim of 'injury' in wrongful life cases is '(i)n essence-...that (defendants), through their negligence, (have) forced upon (the child) the worse of...two alternatives (,)...that nonexistence — never being born — would have been preferable to existence in (the) diseased state....'

"Given this view of the relevant injury which the plaintiff has sustained at the defendant's hands, some courts have concluded that the plaintiff has suffered no legally cognizable injury on the ground that considerations of public policy dictate a conclusion that life — even with the most severe of impairments — is, as a matter of law, always preferable to nonlife. The decisions frequently suggest that a contrary conclusion would 'disavow' the sanctity and value of less-than-perfect human life....

"Although it is easy to understand and to endorse these decisions' desire to affirm the worth and sanctity of less-than-perfect life, we question whether these considerations alone provide a sound basis for rejecting the child's tort action. To begin with, it is hard to see how an award of damages to a severely handicapped or suffering child would 'disavow' the value of life or in any way suggest that the child is not entitled to the full measure of legal and nonlegal rights and privileges accorded to all members of society.

"Moreover, while our society and our legal system unquestionably place the highest value on all human life, we do not think that it is accurate to suggest that this state's public policy establishes—as a matter of law—that under all circumstances 'impaired life' is 'preferable' to 'nonlife.' For example, Health and Safety Code section 7186, enacted in 1968, provides in part: 'The Legislature finds that adult persons have the fundamental right to control the decisions relating to the rendering of their own medical care, including the decision to have life-sustaining procedures withheld or withdrawn in instances of a terminal condition.... The Legislature further finds that, in the interest of protecting individual autonomy, such prolongation of life for persons with a terminal condition may cause loss of patient dignity and unnecessary pain and suffering, while providing nothing medically necessary or beneficial to the patient.' This statute recognizes that—at least in some situations— public policy supports the right of each individual to make his or her own determination as to the relative value of life and death....

"Of course, in the wrongful-life context, the unborn child cannot personally make any choice as to the relative value of life or death. At that stage, however, just as in the case of an infant after birth, the law generally accords the parents the right to act to protect the child's interests. As the wrongful-birth decisions recognize, when a doctor or other medical-care provider negligently fails to diagnose a hereditary problem, parents are deprived of the opportunity to make an informed and meaningful decision whether to conceive and bear a handicapped child.... Although in deciding whether to conceive and bear such a child parents may properly, and undoubtedly do, take into account their own interest, parents also presumptively consider the interests of their future child. Thus, when a defendant negligently fails to diagnose a hereditary ailment, he harms the potential child as well as the parents by depriving the parents of information which may be necessary to determine whether it is in the child's own interest to be born with defects or not to be born at all.

"In this case, in which the plaintiff's only affliction is deafness, it seems quite unlikely that a jury would ever conclude that life with such a condition is worse than not being born at all. Other wrongful-life cases, however, have involved children with much more serious, debilitating and painful conditions, and the academic literature refers to still other, extremely severe hereditary diseases. Considering the short lifespan of many of these children and their frequently very limited ability to perceive or enjoy the benefits of life, we cannot assert with confidence that in every situation there would be a societal consensus that life is preferable to never having been born at all.

"While it thus seems doubtful that a child's claim for general damages should properly be denied on the rationale that the value of impaired life, as a matter of law, always exceeds the value of nonlife, we believe that the out-of-state decisions are on sounder grounds in holding that—with respect to the child's claim for pain and suffering or other general damages—recovery should be denied because (1) it is simply impossible to determine in any rational or reasoned fashion whether the plaintiff has in fact suffered an injury in being born impaired rather than not being born, and (2) even if it were possible to overcome the first hurdle, it would be impossible to assess general damages in any fair nonspeculative manner.

"Judge Weintruab of the New Jersey Supreme Court captured the heart of the problem simply and eloquently in his separate opinion in *Gleitman v. Cosgrove* (1967).... 'Ultimately, the infant's complaint is that he would be better off not to have been born. Man, who knows nothing of death or nothingness, cannot possibly know whether that is so. We must remember that the choice is not being born with health or being born without it.... Rather the choice is between a worldly existence and none at all.... To recognize a right not to be born is to enter an area in which no one can find his way....'

"In responding to this proposition, plaintiff relies on numerous cases which hold that when a defendant has negligently caused a legally cognizable injury, recovery should not totally be denied simply because of the difficulty in ascertaining damages.... She emphasizes that although numerous types of harm—for example, pain and suffering and mental distress—are not readily susceptible to valuation, damages for such items are routinely recoverable in professional malpractice actions, and she argues that if juries are capable of awarding damages for such non-pecuniary harm, they are equally competent to assess appropriate general damages in a wrongful-life case.

"We believe, however, that there is a profound qualitative difference between the difficulties faced by a jury in assessing general damages in a normal personal injury or wrongful-death action, and the task before a jury in assessing general damages in a wrongful-life case. In the first place, the problem is not...simply the fixing of damages for a conceded injury, but the threshold question of determining whether the plaintiff has in fact suffered an injury by being born with an ailment as opposed to not being born at all. As one judge explained: 'When a jury considers the claim of a once-healthy plaintiff that a defendant's negligence harmed him—for example, by breaking his arm—the jury's ability to say that the plaintiff has been 'injured' is manifest, for the value of a healthy existence over an impaired existence is within the experience [or] imagination of most people. The value of nonexistence—its very nature—however, is not....'

"Furthermore, the practical problems are exacerbated when it comes to the matter of arriving at an appropriate award of damages. As already discussed, in fixing damages in a tort case the jury generally compares the condition plaintiff would have been in but for the tort, with the position the plaintiff is in now, compensating the plaintiff for what has been lost as a result of the wrong. Although the valuation of pain and suffering or emotional distress in terms of dollars and cents is unquestionably difficult in an ordinary personal injury action, jurors at least have some frame of reference in their own general experience to appreciate what the plaintiff has lost—normal life without pain and suffering. In a wrongful-life action, that simply is not the case, for what the plaintiff has 'lost' is not life without pain and suffering but rather the unknowable status of never having been born. In this context, a rational, nonspeculative determination of a specific monetary award in accordance with normal tort principles appears to be outside the realm of human competence.

"The difficulty in ascertaining or measuring an appropriate award of general damages in this type of case is also reflected in the application of what is sometimes referred to as the 'benefit' doctrine in tort damages…. '[I]t provides that [w]hen the defendant's tortious conduct has caused harm to the plaintiff…and in so doing has conferred a special benefit to the interest of the plaintiff that was harmed, the value of the benefit conferred is considered in mitigation of damages, to the extent that this is equitable.'

"In requesting general damages in a wrongful-life case, the plaintiff seeks monetary compensation for the pain and suffering he or she will endure because of his or her hereditary affliction. Under [the]…benefit doctrine, however, such damages must be offset by the benefits incidentally conferred by the defendant's conduct 'to the interest of the plaintiff that was harmed.' With respect to general damages, the harmed interest is the child's general physical, emotional and psychological well-being, and in considering the benefit to this interest which defendant's negligence has conferred, it must be recognized that as an incident of defendant's negligence the plaintiff has in fact obtained a physical existence with the capacity both to receive and give love and pleasure as well as to experience pain and suffering. Because of the incalculable nature of both elements of this harm-benefit equation, we believe that a reasoned, nonarbitrary award of general damage is simply not obtainable.

***

"Although we have determined that the trial court properly rejected plaintiff's claim for general damages, we conclude that her claim for the 'extraordinary expenses for specialized teaching, training and hearing equipment' that she will incur during her lifetime because of her deafness stands on a different footing.

***

"Realistically, a defendant's negligence in failing to diagnose a hereditary ailment places a significant medical and financial burden on the whole family unit. Unlike the child's claim for general damages, the damage here is both certain and readily measurable. Furthermore, in many instances these expenses will be vital not only to the child's well-being but to his or her very survival…. If, as alleged, defendants' negligence was in fact a proximate cause of the child's present and continuing need for such special, extraordinary medical care and training, we believe that it is consistent with the basic liability principle of Civil Code section 1714 to hold defendants liable for the cost of such care, whether the expense is to be borne by the parents or by the child....

"Moreover, permitting plaintiff to recover the extraordinary, additional medical expenses that are occasioned by the hereditary ailment is also consistent with the established parameters of the general tort 'benefit' doctrine discussed above. As we have seen, under that doctrine an offset is appropriate only insofar as the defendant's conduct has conferred a special benefit 'to the interest of the plaintiff that was harmed.' Here, the harm for which plaintiff seeks recompense is an economic loss, the extraordinary, out-of-pocket expenses that she will have to bear because of her hereditary ailment. Unlike the claim for general damages, defendants' negligence has conferred no incidental, offsetting benefit to this interest of plaintiff.... Accordingly, assessment of these special damages should pose not unusual or insoluable problems.

"In sum, we conclude that while a plaintiff-child in a wrongful-life action may not recover general damages for being born impaired as opposed to not being born at all, the child—like his or her parents— may recover special damages for the extraordinary expenses necessary to treat the hereditary ailment."

***

(The separate concurring opinion by Justice Newman is deleted.)

JUSTICE MOSK, JOINED BY CHIEF JUSTICE BIRD, DISSENTING:

"I dissent.

"An order is internally inconsistent which permits a child to recover special damages for a so-called wrongful-life action, but denies all general damages for the very same tort. While the modest compassion of the majority may be commendable, they suggest no principle of law that justifies so neatly circumscribing the nature of damages suffered as a result of a defendant's negligence.

***

"I conclude, as did the Court of Appeal in *Curlender*, that a cause of action can be stated and that this handicapped child is entitled to her day in court."

QUESTIONS

1. Is it possible to conclude that nonexistence is preferable to existence? Could one argue that 'wrongful life' is a misnomer? Why isn't it argued that all life is superior to nonexistence?
2. Is the concept of wrongful life merely extreme evidence of a litigious society?
3. How can one measure the damages of a wrongful life?
4. When would a life no longer be considered wrongful? Must a child have a 'serious' defect? When is a defect a 'serious' one? Could not one argue that all lives could be considered wrongful, unless there are some who are born with no physical, mental, or social defects?
5. Is it likely that wrongful-life cases will increase or decrease as medical advances provide us with more information about the fetus in early stages of development?
6. Does *Becker v. Schwartz* and *Turpin v. Sortini* suggest that courts are increasingly willing to allow some damages in such cases? Could it be that the courts are adopting a compromise position in that they recognize that there is some legitimacy to the claim, but remain unwilling to prefer nonexistence to life?

CHAPTER 9

THE RIGHT TO TREATMENT

INTRODUCTION

WITHIN the American legal system, rights can be thought of in two ways: constitutional rights and statutory rights. Constitutional rights are a part of American fundamental law. Statutory rights are those granted by the legislature. A constitutional right is more secure, perhaps because it is a right deeply engrained in the consciousness of the American people. At least a constitutional right is difficult to repeal. A statutory right, on the other hand, is granted by the legislature simply by passing a law, and it can be readily taken away be repealing that law.

There is no general constitutional right to treatment. Although there has been a great deal of litigation over the issue in recent years, the United States Supreme Court has, in a closely divided opinion, stated that there is no such right.[1] At issue was the question of whether the government was obligated to provide free abortions to women unable to afford the costs of an abortion. The Court had previously held that the government had to remove barriers that it had created to the exercise of fundamental rights. However, it stated that it was poverty, rather than a governmentally created barrier, that prevented a woman from getting an abortion. Generally, the government is under no obligation to redress those inequities. Poverty, as a result, may prevent an individual from obtaining desired or even necessary treatment. The Constitution cannot be relied upon to protect the health interests of those unable to pay for medical care.

Statutes, however, can provide a right to treatment. One cannot, for example, be denied treatment at a governmentally funded hospital because of race. There is a statute providing all races the same access to treatment. Similarly, a statute may require governmentally funded hospitals to serve indigents in need of treatment. One problem with such a statutory right, however, has been the lack of clarity of the statute. For the purposes of enforcement of the law, it is important to know what actions are required to place a hospital in com-

---

[1]*Harris v. McRae*, 448 U.S. 297 (1980).

pliance with the law. An enforcement system must also exist to ensure that there is compliance with the law. A statutory right to treatment can be meaningless without specific compliance requirements and adequate enforcement.[2]

In the absence of a constitutional right to treatment or a specific statute providing a right to treatment, there may still be an obligation for health care to be provided those in need of attention. These issues most commonly arise in emergency room denials of admission. Can, for example, a woman in labor be denied admission to a hospital by an emergency room staff member? The judicial response has been mixed, but, absent a specific statute, the courts have often refused to require admission of patients in need.[3]

Another problem in the right to treatment deals with the conflict between patients and the rights of members of the medical community. Suppose, for example, a nurse is morally opposed to abortion. Can that nurse be required to assist in an abortion? One might say that the logical solution would be to assign the nurse to duties where he/she does not have to work with abortion cases. Nurses who are not morally opposed to abortion can assist with abortions. That might be the ideal solution to the problem, but it is not always practical. It may be that all of a hospital's nurses are morally opposed to abortion. If a nurse is needed to assist, either the patient's right to abortion must be denied or a nurse must be compelled to assist. The conflict is not a new one, but it is likely to become increasingly common and is also likely to generate much litigation.[4] Such a conflict is especially likely in abortion cases and sterilization cases. Additionally, one can foresee conflicts developing where members of the medical community have strong feelings over the way the hopelessly ill and dying patient is treated. One may feel that the practice of using extreme measures to prolong life is wrong. Conversely, one may feel that the failure to exert every effort is wrong. Several years ago, at Johns Hopkins Hospital, a Down's syndrome baby was allowed to die. It was inadequately nourished. The baby was in need of surgery to correct a digestive problem, but parental consent to the surgery was denied. That slow process of dying caused moral and emotional

---

[2]For example, see *Newsom v. Vanderbilt University*, 453 F. Supp. 401 (1978).

[3]For example, *Wilmington General Hospital v. Manlove*, 174 A. 2d 135 (1961); *Childs v. Greenville Hospital Authority*, 479 S. W. 2d 399 (1972).

[4]Ramsey, Paul:*Ethics at the Edges of Life* (New Haven, Yale University Press, 1978, pp. 61-77).

anguish to the nursery staff.[5] Here, in a right-to-die case, is another clear example of the conflict between the moral judgments of the staff and the rights of the parents. The court decisions in this area are not settled, but the following cases offer some suggestions over how these conflicts are resolved.

[5]Rachels, James:Euthanasia, killing, and letting die. In Ladd, John (Ed.):*Ethical Issues Relating to Life and Death* (New York, Oxford University Press, 1979, pp. 159-161).

WILMINGTON GENERAL HOSPITAL V. MANLOVE

(Supreme Court of Delaware, 1961)
174 A. 2d 135

Is a hospital liable for the death of an infant whom it refused to treat?

SOUTHERLAND, CHIEF JUSTICE:

∗ ∗ ∗

"On January 4, 1959, Darien E. Manlove, the deceased infant, then four months old, developed diarrhea. The next morning his parents consulted Doctor Hershon. They asked whether the medicine they had for him was all right and the doctor said that it was. In the evening of the same day Mrs. Manlove took the baby's temperature. It was higher than normal. They called Doctor Hershon, and he prescribed additional medication (streptomycin), which he ordered delivered by a pharmacy.

Mrs. Manlove stayed up with the child that night. He did not sleep. On the morning of January 6th the parents took the infant to Doctor Hershon's office. Doctor Thomas examined the child and treated him for sore throat and diarrhea. He prescribed a liquid diet and some medication.

When Mr. Manlove returned home that night, the baby's condition appeared to be the same. His temperature was still above normal, and again he did not sleep during the night.

On the morning of January 7th (a Wednesday) his temperature was still above normal — 102. Mr. and Mrs. Manlove determined to seek additional medical assistance. They knew that Doctor Hershon and Doctor Thomas were not in their offices on Wednesdays, and they took their infant to the emergency ward of the Wilmington General Hospital.

There is no real conflict of fact as to what occurred at the hospital. The parents took the infant into the reception room of the Emergency Ward. A nurse was on duty. They explained to the nurse what was wrong with the child, that is, that he had not slept for two nights, had a continuously high temperature, and that he had diarrhea. Mr. Manlove told the nurse that the child was under the care of Doctor Hershon and Doctor Thomas, and showed the nurse the medicines prescribed. The nurse explained to the parents that the hospital could not give treatment because the child was under the care of a physician and there would be danger that the medication of the hospital might conflict with that of the attending physician. The nurse did not examine the child, take his temperture, feel his forehead, or look down his throat. The child was not in convulsions, and was not coughing or crying. There was no particular area of body tenderness.

The nurse tried to get in touch with Doctor Hershon and Doctor Thomas in the hospital and at their offices, but was unable to do so. She suggested that the parents bring the baby Thursday morning to the pediatric clinic.

Mr. and Mrs. Manlove returned home. Mrs. Manlove made an appointment by telephone to see Doctor Hershon or Doctor Thomas that night at eight o'clock.

At eight minutes past three o'clock in the afternoon the baby died of bronchial pneumonia.

* * *

Plaintiff, as administrator, brought suit against the hospital to recover damages for wrongful death. The complaint charged negligence in failing to render emergency assistance, in failing to examine the baby, in refusing to advise the intern about the child or permit the parents to consult him, and in failing to follow reasonable and humane hospital procedure for the treatment of emergency cases. Defendant answered denying negligence and averring that, pursuant to its established rules and community practice, plaintiff was advised by its employee that it was unable to accept the infant for care.

* * *

The issues made by the parties...were in effect two:

1. Whether the hospital was under any duty to furnish medical treatment to any applicant for it, even in an emergency;
2. Whether the existence of an apparent emergency was a material fact in dispute.

The holding of the court below may be summarized as follows:

1. The hospital is liable for refusal to furnish medical treatment in an emergency because it is a quasi-public institution, being the recipient of grants of public funds and of tax exemptions.

2. There was some evidence of an apparent emergency because
(1) of death following in a few hours, and (2) of the child's
symptoms as recited by the nurse.

We take a somewhat different view of these questions from that
of the learned judge below.

First, as to the status of the defendant hospital.

It was assumed by both parties below that the hospital was a
private hospital and not a public one — that is, an institution founded
and controlled by private persons and not by public authority. The
trial court disagreed, finding a quasi-public status in the receipt of
grants of public money and tax exemptions....

Hence, the court concluded, liability may be imposed on the defendant in an emergency case.

We are compelled to disagree with the view that the defendant
has become a public (or quasi-public) hospital. It is admitted (although the record does not show it) that it is privately owned and
operated. We find no dissent from the rule that such a hospital is a
private hospital, and may, at least in the absence of control by the
legislature, conduct its business largely as it sees fit.

The question of public or private status has frequently arisen in
suits by a physician to compel the hospital to admit him to the use of
its facilities.... The cases uniformly hold that the receipt of public
funds and the exemption from taxation do not convert a private hospital into a public one....

The rule has even been applied to a county-owned hospital if
leased to and operated by a private corporation....

***

Plaintiff attempts to build an argument on 9 Del. C. section
1806, requiring the Levy Court of New Castle County to appropriate $10,000 to the defendant hospital for medical care for indigent
persons suffering from contagious diseases. Subsection (b) provides
that the hospital shall admit and care for such persons.

Plaintiff argues that this is a recognition of the status of the defendant as a public hospital. On the contrary, it is no more than a
condition attached to the gift; or at most a regulation of certain special cases of disease affecting public health. There is no doubt that
medical care is directly related to public health and is therefore an

appropriate subject of legislative regulation; but the provision in subsection (b) only emphasizes the absence of any other provision requiring the hospital to admit anyone.

We are of the opinion that the defendant is a private and not a public hospital, insofar as concerns the right of a member of the public to demand admission or treatment.

What, then is the liability of the hospital in this respect?

Since such an institution as the defendant is privately owned and operated, it would follow logically that its trustees or governing board alone have the right to determine who shall be admitted to it as patients. No other rule would be sensible or workable. Such authority as we have supports this rule.

* * *

We return, then, to the important question: Is there any duty on the part of the hospital to give treatment in an emergency case (i.e. one obviously demanding immediate attention)?

It may be conceded that a private hospital is under no legal obligation to the public to maintain an emergency ward, or, for that matter, a public clinic....

But the maintenance of such a ward to render first-aid to injured persons has become a well-established adjunct to the main business of a hospital. If a person, seriously hurt, applies for such aid at an emergency ward, relying on the established custom to render it, is it still the right of the hospital to turn him away without any reason? In such a case, it seems to us, such a refusal might well result in worsening the condition of the injured person, because of the time lost in a useless attempt to obtain medical aid.

* * *

It must be admitted that there is a dearth of helpful legal precedent. There are very few cases dealing with the liability of a hospital for negligence in connection with the care and treatment of a patient brought to an emergency ward....

The only case cited to us involving refusal of treatment at an emergency ward is that of *O'Neill v. Montefiore Hospital*.... In that case Mr. and Mrs. John J. O'Neill complained of symptoms of a heart ailment or attack. He was refused admission because he was a member of a Hospital Insurance Plan and the hospital did not take such cases. The nurse called an H.I.P. doctor, and Mr. O'Neill took the telephone and described his symptoms. The nurse then arranged for O'Neill to see that doctor a few hours later. Mrs. O'Neill asked to have a doctor examine him because it was an emergency, but this was not done. The O'Neill's returned home, and O'Neill died in a very short time.

In a suit against the doctor and the hospital the trial court found for the defendants. The Appellate Division unanimously reversed as to the doctor. As to the hospital, three judges held there was a question of fact for the jury to decide, that is, whether the nurse's conduct was a personal favor to the deceased, or whether her conduct was that of an attache' discharging her duty, and, if the latter, whether what she did was adequate. Two judges dissented, pointing out that the doctor called by the nurse did not, after talking to the patient, indicate that any emergency treatment was required, or request that the patient be admitted to the hospital. In these circumstances they found no liability.

The difference of opinion in that case seems to turn on the question whether, by calling a physician for the applicant, the nurse assumed to give him hospital service. The case does not discuss the questions of what constitutes an emergency, and what is the duty of the nurse in such cases.

As to the majority holding that the nurse's telephone call gave rise to liability, we respectfully dissent. We think the minority opinion is the better view.

As the above indicated, we are of the opinion that liability on the part of a hospital may be predicated on the refusal of service to a patient in case of an unmistakable emergency, if the patient has relied upon a well-established custom of the hospital to render aid in such a case....

...[W]e inquire, was there an unmistakable emergency? Certainly the record does not support the view that the infant's condition was so desperate that a layman could reasonably say that he was in immediate danger. The learned judge indicated that the fact that death followed in a few hours showed an emergency; but with this we cannot agree. It is hindsight. And it is to be noted that the attending physician, after prescribing for the child on the morning before, did not think another examination that night or the next morning was required. If this case had gone to the jury on the record here made, we would have been required to hold that it was insufficient to establish liability. We cannot agree that the mere recitation of the infant's symptoms was, in itself, evidence of an emergency sufficient to present a question for the jury. Before such an issue could arise there would have to be evidence that an experienced nurse should have known that such symptoms constituted unmistakable evidence of an emergency.

***

We do not think that the record made below satisfactorily developed the pertinent facts....

***

In the circumstances we think the case should go back for further proceedings. We should add, however, that if plaintiff cannot adduce evidence showing some incompetency of the nurse, or some breach of duty or some negligence, his case must fail. Like the learned judge below, we sympathize with the parents in the loss of a child; but this natural feeling does not permit us to find liability in the absence of satisfactory evidence."

***

NEWSOM V. VANDERBILT UNIVERSITY

(U.S. District Court, 1978)

453 F. Supp. 401

To what extent has the Hill-Burton Act provided a right to hospital treatment for indigents?

MORTON, CHIEF JUDGE:

***

"The Hill-Burton Act, one of the earliest forays of the federal government into the health-care field, was enacted in 1946 for the purpose of assisting the states (a) in the development of programs for the construction of facilities for furnishing adequate hospitals, clinics, and similar services to all their people; and (b) to construct public and other nonprofit hospitals in accordance with such programs. Federal money in the form of both grants and loans has been made available under the Act pursuant to plans drawn and administered by the state health agencies with federal approval and supervision.

It is stipulated that (a) Vanderbilt University Hospital received seven federal grants totalling $3,181,009.63 pursuant to the Hill-Burton Act for construction projects initiated between 1957 and 1971; and (b) the receipt of these grants vested the hospital with an obligation to provide a reasonable volume of uncompensated services to persons unable to pay therefor pursuant to the provisions of section 291c(e)(2) of the Act and regulations promulgated thereunder; and (c) in each of the seven applications Vanderbilt gave written assurances that it would provide such services. The manner and extent of Vanderbilt's fulfillment of this obligation and the extent to which the federal and state agencies have monitored and enforced Vanderbilt's compliance are the central issues of this case.

Plaintiff Newsom is an indigent person who contends that the defendant Vanderbilt University's hospital has failed to provide a reasonable volume of services to persons unable to pay therefor in violation of its contractual, statutory and regulatory duties under the Act. She contends in the alternative that even if such services have been provided, the hospital's procedures for the distribution of such care violate procedural due process under the Fifth and Fourteenth Amendments. She further contends that the state and the federal defendants responsible for enforcement of the Act have failed to fulfill that responsibility, and she attacks certain of the federal defendant's regulations as being inconsistent with the Act and the Constitution....

***

HEW's shortcomings in enforcing compliance with the free-care provision of the Hill-Burton Act, attributed by one authority to the tendency of regulatory agencies to become the captive of the veiwpoint of the very interests they were intended to regulate, has created problems in determining just what constitutes compliance. The free-service obligation was virtually ignored until 1972, 25 years after Hill-Burton was enacted and 15 years after Vanderbilt received its first grant. Regulations implementing the free-care obligation in 1947 were 'originally phrased in precatory language, without any provision for enforcement....' The first enforcement regulations were finally promulgated in 1972, but then only after a series of lawsuits forced the agency into action. These regulations have since been changed in several important respects and, in fact, have not yet achieved stability.

The evidence before the court in this case (some of which contradicts the factual bases assigned by the Secretary for his finding of Vanderbilt's compliance) establishes that if the current interpretation of the meaning of 'compliance' were applied retroactively, Vanderbilt would be found seriously wanting. The court agrees that at least until very recently Vanderbilt at best regarded its Hill-Burton obligation as a final write-off for bad debts and at worst ignored it completely....

* * *

It is plaintiff's contention that whether or not Vanderbilt University Hospital has provided a reasonable volume of free services to persons unable to pay, the manner in which it has provided Hill-Burton uncompensated care deprives indigent persons of their rights under the due process provisions of the Fifth and Fourteenth Amendments and violates the Hill-Burton Act. The due process requirements of the Fifth and Fourteenth Amendments may not be imposed upon Vanderbilt unless its allocation of Hill-Burton services constitutes federal and state action.

* * *

On the basis of Vanderbilt's governmental involvement, particularly its administration of its Hill-Burton free-care program, reinforced by its role in thereby performing a state function, this court holds that if the Fifth and Fourteenth Amendments require that due process be provided in the allocation of Hill-Burton free-care, such requirements may be properly imposed upon defendant Vanderbilt. This determination leaves open two questions: first, whether the Fifth and Fourteenth Amendments do in fact require that indigents be afforded due process in the distribution of Hill-Burton free care, and if so, what constitutes due process to such persons.

Defendants argue that because the hospital's obligation is only to provide a reasonable volume of free care, which as a practical matter

in the present case is far short of the need for such care, individual
indigents have no entitlement to such care and are therefore not entitled to due process under the Fifth and Fourteenth Amendments.
Defendants assert in the alternative that the hospital's present procedures, which it alleges conform to the requirements of the statute
and the regulations, provide due process. This court disagrees on
both points.

To determine whether members of the plaintiff class have a constitutionally protected property interest in needed free or below-cost
hospital care, one must look beyond the Constitution itself to other
sources of law, regulations or custom. As the Supreme Court noted
in *Board of Regents v. Roth*..., constitutionally protected property interests 'are created and their dimensions defined by existing rules or
understandings that stem from an independent source such as state
law—rules or understandings that secure certain benefits and that
support claims of entitlements to those benefits....'

Applying the *Roth* directive in this case, it is evident that plaintiff
and the class of indigent persons she represents have a constitutionally protected right to needed uncompensated services under the
Hill-Burton Act. The Act itself defines persons entitled to uncompensated care as being those unable to pay therefor, a statutory
standard of eligibility which the plaintiff class, by definition, meets.
Further definition of the standard was delegated to the states by federal regulation.... Pursuant to such authority, the Tennessee Department of Public Health has developed specific financial eligibility
criteria...which are also satisfied by plaintiff.... In fact, even under
Vanderbilt's own selection practices, such as they are, plaintiff Newsom would have been eligible for uncompensated services.... Thus,
Mrs. Newsom's claim to Hill-Burton uncompensated services is
rooted in both statute and regulation, and constitutes a right en-
forceable by her through the judicial process.... Her claim must,
therefore, be afforded the protections prescribed by the due process
provisions of the Constitution.

This is not to say that plaintiff or other members of the class of
indigent persons have an absolute right to Hill-Burton uncompensated services from defendant Vanderbilt Hospital or from any other
Hill-Burton facility. This right is limited by the extent of the free-
care obligation of Hill-Burton facilities in relation to the need for uncompensated care in their service areas. As in the case of public

assistance payments...limited fiscal resources imply the denial of Hill-Burton benefits to some members of the class of persons unable to pay. But as with welfare, the denial of a right once recognized by statute and regulation can only be effected through procedures conforming with due process requirements to insure that available resources are not allocated arbitrarily....

Having established that members of the plaintiff class have a right to uncompensated care that is protected by the due process provisions of the Fifth and Fourteenth Amendments, it becomes necessary to determine what process is due such persons. This determination must be based on assessment of the nature of public activity that is involved vis-a-vis the private interests implicated in that activity.... In the present case, plaintiff's interest in the fair and consistent allocation of necessary hospital services must be weighed against the defendant hospital's interests in determining eligibility for such services on an *ad hoc* basis, which the record demonstrates has been the case.

There is no disputing the critically important nature of the individual interest here at stake. '[M]edical care is as much a "basic necessity of life" to an indigent as welfare assistance.' The person whose rights are at stake has a need no less brutal than that of a welfare recipient seeking continued public assistance....

The need for procedural regularity in the allocation of Vanderbilt's limited Hill-Burton services is particularly important in light of the unique role played by the hospital in the delivery of care within a large geographic area.... The need for uncompensated care within Davidson County alone far exceeds the amount of Vanderbilt's obligation to provide such care, and many of the patients referred from outlying areas are also indigent. To place this imbalance in its proper context, one must keep in mind that many patients referred to Vanderbilt are sent there because no other facility has the medical resources to treat them.... These medical resources, of course, were developed in part with Hill-Burton subsidies that were allocated to Vanderbilt rather than other facilities in the state.

It is the opinion of this court that due process dictates that indigent persons may be denied necessary medical treatment under the Hill-Burton Act only if they are afforded meaningful notice of their potential eligibility to receive care and of the written eligibility criteria upon which the hospital will base its determination to furnish or withhold treatment. Such persons must also be given timely and adequate written notice detailing the reasons for the proposed denial of benefits, review by a decision-maker who has not participated in making the initial finding of ineligibility, and a written statement of the reasons for the decision and the evidence relied on.... At the core of due process is of course a requirement that individuals be given an effective opportunity to present affirmative evidence and to refute adverse evidence, though not necessarily at an oral hearing....

These procedures can be accommodated to the need, shared by patient and hospital alike, for prompt processing of requests for treatment. Vanderbilt already utilizes a process of screening prospective patients for the purpose of restricting indigent admissions. This process could be modified without major cost or inconvenience to the hospital to insure that the facility provides a reasonable volume of Hill-Burton care as required, and to provide the necessary constitutional protection to persons denied such care....

The procedural protections set forth above...are not only required by the Constitution but are necessary to the fulfillment of the purposes of the Hill-Burton Act itself. Unless an indigent person is afforded an opportunity to know what substantive criteria are being used to determine whether he will receive some of the limited Hill-Burton benefits, it is impossible for him—or for regulatory authorities—to assure that his demand for needed services has been accorded fair treatment. Without written, published standards, the personal biases and predilections of individual hospital staff could serve as the bases for denial of needed uncompensated services under the Act. An opportunity to be heard would be meaningless, since in the absence of predetermined criteria, the indigent person's objections to a denial of care could be answered simply by an *ad hoc* revision of the reasons for the denial.

***

...The primary differences in the present procedure and the procedure required by the due process clauses are (1) Vanderbilt currently 'reviews' only those cases that have been approved by the lower decision-maker, and (2) the patient receives little if any information concerning the decision process or the decision itself. In fact he may never know he was considered for Hill-Burton free care at all. For anyone to contend that such treatment constitutes due process borders on the absurd.

* * *

"...Defendant Vanderbilt is hereby enjoined from reporting services as Hill-Burton uncompensated care unless such services qualify and are shown by the hospital's records to qualify under the Act and current regulations, and it is enjoined from reporting Hill-Burton uncompensated care on any basis other than that prescribed to the Act or current regulations promulgated under the Act. Defendant Vanderbilt is further enjoined from bringing, or having brought on its behalf, an action to collect amounts owed by any patient for services that would have qualified as Hill-Burton care but for the improper acts of defendant hospital. The state and federal defendants are enjoined from finding Vanderbilt to be in compliance with its free-care obligation on the basis of reports and/or hospital records that do not clearly evidence compliance under the Act and current regulations."

* * *

WOLFE V. SCHROERING

(U.S. District Court, 1974)
388 F. Supp. 631

Is a state law constitutional that allows public hospitals to refuse to perform abortions?

BRATCHER, DISTRICT JUDGE:

* * *

"This is a class action seeking declaratory and injunctive relief against the enforcement of the provisions of the recently-enacted Kentucky Abortion Statute, Senate Bill No. 259. Plaintiffs vigorously contend that the overriding purpose and dominant effect of the Statute under attack is to discourage and interfere with certain clearly defined, constitutionally protected rights of the plaintiffs....

* * *

"In the wake of the Supreme Court decisions of *Roe v. Wade*...and *Doe v. Bolton*...the Kentucky General Assembly in the 1974 legislative session enacted Senate Bill No. 259 entitled "An Act Relating to the Regulation of Abortion," which became effective June 21, 1974. It consists of nineteen sections....

* * *

"This Court cannot romp about capriciously in this matter but is obliged to examine the subject legislation in light of the mandate of the Supreme Court.... Even though tedious and time-consuming, we will take a section-by-section approach and inspect each questioned provision.

* * *

"Section 11. This section deals with the state not requiring hospitals to perform abortions and an anti-discrimination clause for hospitals that choose not to perform abortions. This section is challenged in itself and in relation to Section 6(2) which requires that all post-first trimester abortions be performed in a hospital or clinic meeting certain minimal requirements.

"This Court believes that the Section 11 and Section 6(2) regulations are unconstitutional in that they single out abortions, thereby treating the abortion process differently from other medical procedures. *Nyberg v. City of Virginia*...clearly holds that a public hospital 'may not arbitrarily preclude abortions from the variety of services offered which require no greater expenditure of available facilities and skills....' In order to comply with the constitutional principles set out in *Roe* and *Doe*, the state cannot allow a public hospital to refuse to perform abortions as a policy. Further, the state cannot subtly discourage the performing of abortions by providing that hospitals which do not allow abotions may not be discriminated against when no such provision exists for hospitals which do perform abortions.

"The Court finds no objection with Section 6(2) standing alone. While Sections 11 and 6(2) together were tainted with an unconstitutional effect, without Section 11, Section 6(2) does not violate the Constitution."

* * *

HARRIS V. McRAE

(U.S. Supreme Court, 1980)
448 U.S. 297

Must the government provide free abortions to those unable to pay?

JUSTICE STEWART:

* * *

"Since September, 1976, Congress has prohibited—either by an amendment to the annual appropriations bill for the Department of Health, Education, and Welfare or by a joint resolution—the use of any federal funds to reimburse the cost of abortions under the Medicaid program except under certain specified circumstances. This funding restriction is commonly known as the 'Hyde Amendment,' after its original congressional sponsor, Representative Hyde. The current version of the Hyde Amendment, applicable for fiscal year 1980, provides: '(N)one of the funds provided by this joint resolution shall be used to perform abortions except where the life of the mother would be endangered if the fetus were carried to term; or except for such medical procedures necessary for the victims of rape or incest when such rape or incest has been reported promptly to a law enforcement agency or public health service....' This version of the Hyde Amendment is broader than that applicable for fiscal year 1977, which did not include the 'rape or incest' exception..., but narrower than that applicable for most of fiscal year 1978, and all of fiscal year 1979, which had an additional exception for 'instances where severe and long-lasting physical health damage to the mother would result if the pregnancy were carried to term when so determined by two physicians....'

* * *

"The Hyde Amendment...places no governmental obstacle in the path of a woman who chooses to terminate her pregnancy, but rather, by means of unequal subsidization of abortion and other medical services, encourages alternative activity deemed in the public interest....

"It is evident that a woman's interest in protecting her health was an important theme in *Wade*. In concluding that the freedom of a woman to decide whether to terminate her pregnancy falls within the personal liberty protected by the Due Process Clause, the Court in *Wade* emphasized the fact that the woman's decision carries with it significant personal health implications—both physical and psychological....

"But, regardless of whether the freedom of a woman to choose to terminate her pregnancy for health reasons lies at the core or the periphery of the due process liberty recognized in *Wade*, it simply does not follow that a woman's freedom of choice carries with it a constitutional entitlement to the financial resources to avail herself of the full range of protected choices. The reason...: although government may not place obstacles in the path of a woman's exercise of her freedom of choice, it need not remove those not of its own creation. Indigency falls in the latter category. The financial constraints that restrict an indigent woman's ability to enjoy the full range of constitutionally protected freedom of choice are the product not of governmental restrictions on access to abortion, but rather on her indigency. Although Congress has opted to subsidize medically necessary services generally, but not certain medically necessary abortions, the fact remains that the Hyde Amendment leaves an indigent woman with at least the same range of choice in deciding whether to obtain a medically necessary abortion as she would have had if Congress had chosen to subsidize no health-care costs at all. We are thus persuaded that the Hyde Amendment impinges on the constitutionally protected freedom of choice recognized in *Wade*.

* * *

...."[T]he principle impact of the Hyde Amendment falls on the indigent. But the fact does not itself render the funding restriction constitutionally invalid, for this Court has held repeatedly that poverty, standing alone, is not a suspect classification....

* * *

"Where, as here, the Congress has neither invaded a substantive constitutional right or freedom, nor enacted legislation that purposefully operates to the detriment of a suspect class, the only requirement of equal protection is that congressional action be rationally related to a legitimate governmental interest. The Hyde Amendment satisfies that standard. It is not the mission of this Court or any other to decide whether the balance of competing interests reflected in the Hyde Amendment is wise social policy. If that were our mission, not every Justice who has subscribed to the judgment of the Court today could have done so. But we cannot, in the name of the Constitution, overturn duly enacted statutes simply 'because they may be unwise, improvident, or out of harmony with a particular school of thought....' Rather, 'when an issue involves policy choices as sensitive as those implicated [here]..., the appropriate forum for their resolution in a democracy is the legislature....' "

* * *

MR. JUSTICE BRENNAN, WITH WHOM MR. JUSTICE MARSHALL AND MR. JUSTICE BLACKMAN JOIN, DISSENTING:

"...[T]he State's interest in protecting the potential life of the fetus cannot justify the exclusion of financially and medically needy women from the benefits to which they would otherwise be entitled solely because the treatment that a doctor has concluded is medically necessary involves an abortion....

* * *

"When viewed in the context of the Medicaid program to which it is appended, it is obvious that the Hyde Amendment in nothing less than an attempt by Congress to circumvent the dictates of the Constitution and achieve indirectly what *Roe v. Wade* said it could not do directly.... [T]he Hyde Amendment is a transparent attempt by the Legislative Branch to impose the political majority's judgment of the morally acceptable and socially desirable preference on a sensitive and intimate decision that the Constitution entrusts to the individual. Worse yet, the Hyde Amendment does not force that majoritarian viewpoint with equal measure upon everyone in our Nation, rich and poor alike; rather, it imposes that viewpoint only upon that segment of our society which, because of its position of political powerlessness, is least able to defend its privacy rights from the encroachments of state-mandated morality. The instant legislation thus calls for more exacting judicial review than in most other cases. 'When elected leaders cower before public pressure, this Court, more than ever, must not shirk its duty to enforce the Constitution for the benefit of the poor and powerless....'

"Moreover, it is clear that the Hyde Amendment not only was designed to inhibit, but does in fact inhibit the woman's freedom to choose abortion over childbirth.... In every pregnancy, one of these two courses of treatment is medically necessary, and the poverty-stricken woman depends on the Medicaid Act to pay for the expenses associated with that procedure. But under the Hyde

Amendment, the Government will fund only those procedures incidental to childbirth. By thus injecting coercive financial incentives favoring childbirth into a decision that is constitutionally guaranteed to be free from governmental intrusion, the Hyde Amendment deprives the indigent woman of her freedom to choose abortion over maternity, thereby impinging on the due process liberty right recognized in *Roe v. Wade*."

* * *

(The separate concurring opinion by Justice White is deleted. The separate dissents by Justices Marshall, Stevens and Blackman are also deleted.)

QUESTIONS

1. Has the state by enacting a conscience clause improperly burdened the right to an abortion? If no physician in a community was willing to perform abortions, could they be forced to do so against their will?
2. Would a taxpayer conscience clause, in which taxpayers who were opposed to abortion forbade their tax monies' use for providing free abortions, be unconstitutional?
3. Why isn't the right to health care a fundamental constitutional right? Should it be?
4. Was a right to health care established in Hill-Burton which is the equivalent of a constitutional right to health care?
5. May a physician or hospital refuse to care for an indigent patient in desperate need of health care?
6. What is the government's obligation to correct economic inequalities in health care?
7. How extensive an effort should be made to provide health care to those unable to pay? Should, for example, the government pay for free heart transplants?

INDEX

259